Unstoppable

A Personal Trainer's Guide to Business Success

Jared Garcia

Unstoppable: A Personal Trainer's Guide to Business Success
Success
By Jared Garcia

Copyright © 2017 by Jared Garcia

Printed and bound in the United States of America

ISBN: 978-1-98-129189-2

Acknowledgements

To Noleen Arendse for her editorial insights, strong work ethic, and focus on building a complete story. Though she worked halfway across the world, her communication and strength helped carry this manuscript to its final form. Words cannot describe how appreciative I am of her work.

To Pierre Tapia for inspiring the book and his relentless motivation throughout the writing process. His consistent feedback, energy and friendship helped bring this book to the world.

Dedication

This book is dedicated to my parents, Lisa and Manuel, who have supported me through all my crazy adventures. I thank you for your unwavering love and support.

Table of Contents

Preface

I deeply understand the problems of the personal training role, whether you're a prospective personal trainer, an intermediate trainer, or currently excelling; I've been there personally.

I have a degree in Exercise Biology (aka Kinesiology). I have a number of certifications including NSCA-CSCS (National Strength and Conditioning Association - Certified Strength and Conditioning Specialist), TRX, Z-Health, CHEK Holistic Lifestyle Coach, Functional Movement System (FMS), and USA Weightlifting. I've been around and learned from hundreds of personal trainers in different stages of their career and knowledge. I've seen hundreds of clients with varying backgrounds, personalities, goals, values, and motivations — I've trained for years. I know how difficult it is to start as a personal trainer; to answer the call. I know how much experience it takes to reach a level that you're comfortable with financially, psychologically, and emotionally.

In addition to the certifications and my bachelor's degree, I've opened my own independent training business and I've worked at big box gyms in San Francisco, including Equinox. I've also designed, prototyped and built my own fitness products, and consulted on fitness software. I've trained millionaires and billionaires, as well as clients who understand the science and would prod me with questions around how the different body systems interact during exercise. I've trained elite athletes who understand the very specific niche exercises and clients new to exercise who have general goals (i.e. weight loss, diet transitioning). And, like any other experienced personal trainer, I've trained many clients with varying temperaments. I've had to balance these clients against my own personality and daily stressors, with much success.

Why do I tell you about my background? I tell you because I know what it's like to be where you are in your career, finances, experience, and knowledge. I also know I have a deep passion for fitness and helping people succeed. And I know that if you are thinking about joining, or growing in this industry, you have something similar inside yourself. You have a deep intrinsic desire to help people reach their goals, and that should be valued and nurtured.

If you're reading this book, then you already have the awareness that you want to better your professional career, which will trickle down into all other aspects of your life. You want to improve your life, and I can completely relate because I've had the same feeling inside me. As a personal trainer, I was working so much, running around from client to client, exploring different avenues for success, trying different sales and marketing techniques; using so much time and effort, and wanting to do better — yet not knowing how to do that. And I know there are many of you reading this book that are going through the same situations. You question if you really have what it takes to succeed. You ask yourself if personal training was a good career choice, a good life path.

If you have the passion to continue in this industry, keep reading. Throughout this book, I'll provide you with the knowledge gained from years of experience, highlighted through specific activities and stories designed to inspire and educate you on your path to success. Unstoppable is intended to be a book that changes your thinking and your view of the profession of personal training. Every chapter is loaded with practical content that will bring value to your career as a personal trainer and to your business. There's also the opportunity to learn more, with VIP access to online bonus content. I encourage you to use this book as a resource to come back to again and again as your business grows.

Keep reading and discover how to become a successful personal trainer.

The Dream — The Reality

He was on the edge, the cliff dropped away suddenly. Luke found himself teetering forward, the magnetism of the height drawing him closer... he reached out expecting to have a free hand but found his hands full. For some reason, he had a pile of his grandma's treasured china plates in both hands, he was trying to balance... trying to hold up the plates... he wobbled and felt himself falling...

Luke woke up in a sweat. He had that sick feeling in his gut from too little sleep. He dragged himself out of bed, it was 4 a.m. He'd only climbed into bed after midnight, and his sleep was once more restless and anxious. He had to meet his first personal training client at five. The client was a busy executive who got going early in the morning to beat the competition. Luke grabbed his gym bag and dashed out of his apartment.

He arrived at the gym just before his client. His boss, Kirsten, was getting the reception desk ready for the day. "Hey Luke, pretty early today. You're looking rugged... rough night?" Luke gave a smile, a weak one which quickly changed to a mask of professionalism as his client came in through the door. "Hey, Luke. I'm in a rush today, I've got a flight to catch." His client dashed past with an air of importance into the locker room.

Luke started up the stairs to the gym floor. As his hand touched the banister, he thought back to the first time he climbed those stairs. He had literally run up the stairs that day, but today his feet felt like lead. He remembered the excitement, the smells — bleach, rubber mats, sweat, and protein-shake — it was his first day as an assistant.

While he was still in his senior year at college, his career guidance counselor had recommended that he work at the local gym part-time. Luke had always been interested in fitness. He was one of those guys that naturally gravitated towards athletics. He loved it and lived it. He was passionate about fitness and that passion overflowed into helping others around him. He helped his friends improve their physical fitness and encouraged his family to live healthy, active lives. He modeled this to them and his example inspired them. It only made sense that after college he would become a personal trainer. So, during the summer break, Luke had applied to Kirsten's gym to work as an assistant. She had been impressed by his attitude to fitness, health, and life. She had seen potential in him and had gladly asked him to join her team.

The smell of his client's cologne jolted him back to reality. "Hi John, how are you doing today? What time's your flight?" Luke ushered his client to the treadmill to begin their warm-up. "Doing well Luke, it's going to be a busy one. My flight is at nine, so I'll have to cut it short today. I'm working on this huge deal..." John started talking, and Luke's attention drifted. He looked across the gym and saw a flash of the back of a personal trainer's top. It triggered a vivid memory...

When he was an assistant, he would watch the personal trainers — he saw them as the legends in the gym — the guys who had "made it." While he was helping yet another gym-goer use the step-machine, he would watch the PTs with their clients. They would be on the floor wearing their tops with "Personal Trainer" written across the back. They always seemed to be in control, they appeared successful. They could come and go as they pleased, work their own hours, be their own boss. Luke dreamed of being just like them. No more stacking weights, cleaning equipment and picking up after the guys on the weight floor for a pittance. He would become a legend too, he would make more money and be a successful trainer, he would make a difference in his clients' lives, maybe he would even become a celebrity trainer... that had been the dream...

"Hey, Luke?!" It was John, "I've been walking for 10 minutes. Let's get going, man..." Luke managed to focus through the rest of the session. Because his client had to leave early, Luke followed the cookie-cutter routine. Treadmill warm-up... weights... stretch. His client didn't really need that type of routine, but it was easy and Luke didn't have to think too much. His client saw him as an accessory in any case... every exec has a personal trainer... it's "in."

Luke sighed, he felt empty and unfulfilled. When he first became a personal trainer, he had such hopes of changing people's lives. He had received his certification and, Kirsten, impressed by his determination, his passion, and his work ethic, had offered him a position as a personal trainer. He had been confident that he would make it. However, a couple of months into working and Luke's dream began to fade — rapidly. His hope of being a "legend" and "making it" faded even faster. He found that the clients didn't just flock to him because he was "certified." He had to work long hours to fit in as many clients as possible just to make ends meet. He got home exhausted at night, having had too much coffee, eaten junk and not trained himself. His dreams of having loads of money, transformed into loads of dirty gym clothes. Luke found himself juggling so many things, like those plates in his dream, and although he knew how to train his clients, he didn't know how to turn that into a successful business.

Luke, feeling exhausted, sat in the canteen and stared aimlessly into the gym. Working those crazy hours and trying to see as many clients as possible was not making him more successful, in fact, instead of feeling motivated, energized and ready to help, he was feeling drained, depressed and unmotivated — and he wasn't making money, he was just getting by. He knew that he couldn't carry on in his current state, he was most definitely on the edge of that cliff ... a crisis point.

Introduction

If you've worked as a personal trainer, or have known someone who is involved in personal training, then you will be familiar with Luke's story or aspects of his story. I know I can, I've been there.

I studied physical therapy and started personal training in college. Over a period of four years, I worked in multiple environments, from large gyms to small, sports teams to individual clients. I gained much knowledge and experience in those various fields and did well with many aspects of personal training. Yet, I found myself needing to juggle multiple tasks and skills, and I lacked the knowledge on how to integrate them and focus them into operating a successful business. I felt as if I was missing something and not reaching my full potential. I didn't know how to fix the issues.

Some of you reading this book will be able to relate to what I was feeling. You want to *be* better, to *do* better, you want to succeed — but don't know how to do that. You have all the head knowledge to train people, the certification that says you that can train people, but find that you lack the actual skills to turn that into a successful business. You question if you really have what it takes to succeed. You ask yourself if personal training was a good career choice; a good life path. If this feels like you, keep reading. The knowledge and the tools to become successful as a personal trainer are here — in this book.

It took me years to figure out how to put it altogether and into a successful business model. I understand where many personal trainers find themselves — and that's why I wrote this book. The aim is to fast-track your learning curve and pathway to success.

In your hands, you will find all the information and resources that you need to become successful in personal training. You will learn to focus your knowledge, your attention and your desire to bring value to your clients. You will be equipped with all the tools that you need and I will help you integrate them into your daily life using hands-on application activities. I encourage you to do them — don't skip the activities. It's in the *doing* that you will learn and grow; the *doing* will boost you on your way to success.

But this is just the beginning, http://www.MakeMoney PersonalTraining.com has loads of resources that will continue to inspire you on your journey.

You *can* make more than a living wage and can be successful at personal training. There are so many niches and opportunities into which you can expand your profession — with a little creativity, passion, and using and applying what you learn in this book — you can become successful.

This book is not just another "how-to-book," it's about you and your journey to becoming a successful personal trainer. I've been on this journey, and my goal is to help you on yours.

Chapter One

The World of Personal Training

So, let's start at the beginning. Let's review the world of personal training.

What is Personal Training?

Wikipedia defines the role of a personal trainer as an individual who has a varying degree of knowledge of general fitness involved in exercise prescription and instruction. To the outside world, we — personal trainers — bring exercise and fitness into the daily lives of our clients. We are hired to integrate these fitness programs into our clients' hectic schedules.

However, within the personal trainer community, we know ourselves to be more than just "bringers of fitness." We are individuals who care for our clients on a daily, monthly and yearly basis. We are integrators of health, facilitators of healthy activities; we coach, we counsel, we encourage, we cheer, we are motivators — we are life changers.

Why Become a Personal Trainer?

There are many reasons why people become personal trainers. Here are some of the more popular ones that I've encountered:

- I'm good at working out
- I used to be an athlete
- I know how the body works

- I've taken a few science or anatomy classes
- I have family in the health industry
- I love sports, fitness, or exercise
- I want to make money; this seems easy
- I'm good at selling fitness stuff
- I have passion for the personal training role

As you can see, the *why's* vary from person to person. Later on, we will be looking at this in a bit more detail because your *why* plays an integral role in determining your pathway to success.

What do People Generally Believe About Personal Training?

Our view of life is formed by what we believe. When we have an incorrect belief about something, it limits us and limits our journey to success.

There are many incorrect beliefs about personal trainers. These misconceptions are held by those outside the fitness world, and from inside the fitness industry — sometimes, even by personal trainers themselves.

Let's look at some of the incorrect beliefs held by the general public, and encouraged by television, movies and social media:

- Personal trainers are just interested in exercise; they only care about the physical aspects of life — namely fitness.
- Personal trainers are unintelligent, uneducated and are "meat-heads."
- Personal trainers have taken the "easy route." They want to make a quick buck without getting a "normal" job.
- Personal trainers don't really make a difference to people's lives.
- Personal trainers are "just a craze." They are "in" because all celebrities have PT's and therefore to be "in" you must have one.

These are just a few of the misconceptions, but you can see that most of them are held because of a lack of education about the profession of personal training and the value that we can bring. And here is a key:

When you believe and know you can bring value, and you bring value to a client, you will be on the pathway to success

Unfortunately, personal trainers themselves have some incorrect beliefs about personal training, which will limit their thinking. Beliefs such as...

Health professionals respect our certification, our fitness philosophies and health advice:

There are a few health professionals that do respect our certifications, however, the majority have the same misconceptions as the general public because they have not been educated otherwise. We'll touch on this a bit later, but there is an untapped market in partnering with non-fitness health professionals such as doctors, chiropractors, dieticians and physiotherapists. It's up to us to educate them otherwise and to show them the value that we can bring to our clients.

Our clients will listen to us because we've spent years educating ourselves on health topics, and we can show them the latest health and fitness trends — which they care about and want to follow:

This isn't true. From my experience, I have found that most clients are not interested in the latest hyped-up fitness trend. Some are not even keen to try it and feel embarrassed to do so. Our clients want their needs met. They want results and they want to achieve those results in a way that is customized to their personal preferences and lifestyle.

We don't have to sell or market ourselves — because we are personal trainers, the clients will come:

We believe clients will buy what we're selling just because *we're* selling it. We, as personal trainers, have a "build it, and they will come" mindset. *Wrong.* Personal trainers should sell all the time and market our services appropriately. We'll be showing you *how* later on — so keep reading.

In the fitness world, having a certification means you are "skilled" and "equipped" to be a personal trainer:

In the fitness community, we believe that having a certification means somebody is a good (-enough) personal trainer. We also believe *not* having a certification means somebody is not worthy of being a personal trainer. We'll be looking at certifications later — but from my experience, just because you have a certification (and it does help), it does not mean you will be a successful personal trainer.

In the fitness world, your rate per hour, your work venue and your workload determines your success.

The industry believes that if you're personal training at a lower session rate per hour, you're not as good a personal trainer as somebody with a higher per session rate. If you don't work at a big gym, you're not going to make it. Our industry believes if you don't have a few years of experience, or your schedule isn't currently filled with clients — you're not going to be successful.

However, as you journey through this book, you will find that these factors don't determine your success. There is a saying by Wayne Dyer that goes: *"If you change the way you look at things, the things you look at change."* We'll be changing our views of personal training and success. Which leads us to the next question...

What do We Mean by Being a "Successful" Personal Trainer?

As we mentioned, everyone will have their own reasons for

becoming a personal trainer and each one will also have their own definition of "success." *What is your definition of success as a personal trainer?*

For me, a business should be profitable and sustainable. My personal cutoff for financial success is a six-figure income. Currently, in the fitness industry, the median salary for personal trainers is approximately $57,000 per year. Additionally, almost 50% of personal trainers have only one to four years of experience, which means they don't last long in the industry. Based on these stats, currently, in the fitness industry, only 1–5% of personal trainers are successful. Or in other words, 95–99% of personal trainers don't reach their full potential in the industry.

So Why Do Personal Trainers Fail?

To cover all the reasons why personal trainers fail would be a book in itself. In this book, we will be focusing on the gap between the theory and the actual skills required to run a successful personal training business and why this gap causes many to fail. We will also be bridging that gap for you. So, you may be asking, "What do you mean by 'gap'?" Let me explain...

Contrary to widely held belief, the profession of personal training is far more involved than "just prescribing exercise." It is a multi-faceted profession and to be successful we, as personal trainers, need to learn how to integrate our skills, tools and knowledge, including bringing all our deepest passions as fitness professionals and health integrators into personalized, successful packages to our clients. Not only that, but we also need to learn how to integrate and balance the many tasks and activities involved in running a business. From sales and marketing, to accounts and administrative tasks, to customizing exercise programs and eating plans — there is a lot to balance and master — and very few certification programs will teach you the actual "how-to's" of integrating all those skills, tools and knowledge into a well-functioning business.

The best certifications are effective at teaching science, program design, and running a session. And only a few certification bodies give advice on sales, business basics, and information on the industry. And, although personal trainers are certified, we only get trained in a few of these skills and are then sent out into the world to fend for ourselves. Our industry and certifications are not effective in producing personal trainers that are equipped to integrate all the tools and skills into a balanced, well-functioning, fulfilling and financially successful long-term business.

That's why you will find that most personal trainers are usually only good at one or two aspects of personal training, whether it's sales, marketing, personal passion, the psychology of a client, the science background, developing a program, industry knowledge, or running a client session. Most trainers will have unbalanced skills — they are good in one area, but lack skill in the other aspects necessary for success. It is not often that you will find a personal trainer that is balanced in all those areas, and you will rarely encounter a personal trainer set up for present and future success.

You may be thinking, "What's so wrong with being unbalanced?" Well, in the same way that a muscle imbalance will impact on a person's ability to perform and reach their full potential, so too will a lack of balanced and integrated skills prevent a personal trainer from reaching their full potential. A personal trainer who doesn't reach their full potential (personal, financial, professional) will feel a lack within themselves — they'll feel as if they aren't giving enough to their clients, they may feel regret for not achieving their professional goals or shame for not reaching their financial aspirations. A client with an unbalanced personal trainer may also feel burdened — they could feel taken advantage of (through hard-selling, false advertising), they may feel there's too much focus on fitness and nutritional science, or the program is too idealistic and doesn't integrate into their normal life.

Additionally, present success doesn't guarantee future success. The industry is constantly changing with shifts in technology, psychology, training methods, and fads. To achieve success, we need to be ahead of the curve. Most personal trainers rely too heavily on a few developed skills, get industry tunnel-vision, and don't change fast enough to accommodate for the future. When personal trainers don't accommodate to the changing industry, it leads to less success for their clients, their business, and ultimately less success for themselves.

As I mentioned in the beginning of the book, I can personally relate to the state of the unbalanced personal trainer because I've been there. After a few years of personal training, I had gained much experience, yet, I was still unbalanced. When I first became a personal trainer, I didn't select a niche, I was not confident in sales techniques, and I disliked marketing. I felt like there was a gap in my ability, despite having a certification and a great deal of scientific knowledge. It took me years to gather the unfocused tools from the various certifications and integrate them into a successful system, which I have now made available to you.

Why Does This Matter to You?

As a new personal trainer, or an experienced trainer who isn't reaching their full potential, it's crucial to understand this knowledge gap and the impact that it can have on your success. Most trainers don't understand the cause of the issues and how to fix them, so the problem compounds itself leading to unmet professional and financial dreams by the end of their career. There are hundreds of thousands of personal trainers in the US alone and more throughout the rest of world. Each one of you can be a successful personal trainer if you're primed with the knowledge of *how* to be successful. Additionally, our clients and prospects care more and more about health, nutrition, and fitness each year. The need for a personal trainer is around you. There are enough people who request fitness services and want to experience living healthy lives daily, but need someone to bridge the gap between the sheer amount of information on health and fitness, and applying it to their very busy lives. And that's where we succeed — we build this bridge with our clients, we take the massive amount of health knowledge and focus it for the betterment of our clientele and bring value into their lives.

We bridge the health gap for our clients and now it's time to bridge the gap for your personal success. We are going to take the massive amount of knowledge and skills that you do have and focus them. Having focused knowledge can lend itself to more freedom in your schedule, whether that's starting at (or launching!) a gym, becoming an independent contractor, or working in any other personal training capacity.

The objective of this book is to lay out a clear path between the theory of personal training and the actual skills required to become successful as a personal trainer. As you follow the path, you will save time because everything you need to start off as a personal trainer, and to succeed — is right here.

I encourage you to keep reading and to *apply* all the activities. In doing so, you will be equipped to achieve your financial and professional goals. Goals such as: earning more money, working normal hours (8 a.m. to 6 p.m.), increasing your per session price, only working with clients you enjoy, increasing your knowledge and skills, being happy, experiencing financial freedom, schedule flexibility, opening a gym and being your own boss.

Chapter Two

Finding Your "Why"

"If your why is strong enough, you'll figure out the how."
- Bill Walsh –

The sound of the canteen chair being scraped back, cut in on Luke's slump. It was Kirsten. "Can I join you?" She put her coffee cup on the table. "Looks like it's been a rough day for you. How are you really doing, Luke?"

Kirsten was a great boss. She always took the time to check up on her trainers. Over the last couple of months, Luke had been so busy that she hadn't been able to connect with him. She had noticed him losing weight, and not in a good way. She had also noticed the spark of passion fading. He used to bounce into the gym, ready for his clients. He would take the time to build great relationships with them and would tailor his programs especially to their likes and dislikes. He wanted them to enjoy their sessions. But, lately, she had observed his sessions becoming more routine. Planned, but not as well thought out as they used to be. She had seen Luke drifting off somewhere in his mind when training his clients — he would take on a vacant look and not really pay attention to them in the way that he used to. His client numbers were also dropping; he had lost quite a few clients in the last month or so, and soon she would need to warn him that she would have to let him go, something that she didn't want to do. Kirsten was worried...

Luke shook his head and sighed. He didn't normally talk about how he was doing, but today it came tumbling out, "*Why* did I get into personal training? What was I thinking? I'm feeling totally overwhelmed. I know I have these skills and I can train clients... but I'm feeling frustrated that I don't know how to put it all together. I've been having dreams of juggling precious china on the edge of a precipice, and that's what I feel like I'm doing. I'm juggling so many things, trying to cope, trying to succeed... but all the while feeling like I'm looming over a gap, constantly on the edge of failure. I see my hopes and dreams of being successful, of making a difference in people's lives, but between myself and that success is this gap and I don't know how to bridge it. For the first time, I feel like quitting... just walking away."

Kirsten sighed and nodded her head. She could totally relate to him. She had been in a similar place before and her good friend, Ted, had given her a helping hand. He had journeyed with her, mentored her and helped her become a successful personal trainer, and now a gym owner. Ted had showed her how to take the theory, the tools and the skills, and integrate them into becoming successful as a personal trainer *and* in the business of personal training.

Ted had recently had a car accident and injured his legs quite severely. He owned a thriving gym in a different niche to Kirsten. He was a very "hands-on" type of gym owner and now, because of the car accident, he was needing someone to be an extra set of hands. Maybe Kirsten could help him — and Luke.

"You know, Luke, one of the first things that I noticed in you was your desire to help people — your *why* is because you genuinely want to make a difference in people's lives. It was because of that passion that I gave you the position. Being a personal trainer is tough; it takes a long time to work out how to put it altogether and to find your feet. When I found myself on that precipice, I was blessed enough to have someone give me a helping hand and show me how to do just that, put it altogether." Luke looked up, he was listening. Kirsten continued, "I think I can help you. My friend, Ted, runs a very successful gym across town. He's a great guy and loves working with his clients. Unfortunately, he was in a motor vehicle accident recently — he injured his legs and is on crutches for a couple of months. He is looking for someone to come in and be an extra set of hands for him. He needs someone who is passionate about helping people, to train his clients. The pay will be good and the clients are consistent. I think you will be a great fit." She slid a business card across the table, "Luke, I know you feel like quitting right now. But, just give this a try. He only needs someone for a couple of months. If, after those months, you still want to quit... then go for it. At least you will have explored it and can make a better decision as to where you want to go career-wise."

Luke put the card in his wallet, "Thanks, Kirsten. I'll give it some thought. I appreciate you listening to me." He picked up his bag and got ready to leave.

"You're welcome, Luke... and Luke, get some sleep tonight." She gave him a hug, "I really hope you'll give Ted a call in the morning. I'll message him to say that I might have a potential contact."

That night, Luke crawled into bed early. He put his wallet next to his bed, and the card fell out. He picked it up and read, *"Transform your life - Personal Training and Lifestyle Coaching."* He decided to call Ted in the morning.

***

> "If you can't figure out your purpose, figure out your passion. For your passion will lead you right into your purpose."
> -Bishop TD Jakes-

If you're reading this book, then you already have the awareness that you want to better your life professionally, and if you are a new personal trainer, you most likely have a deep desire to succeed and make a difference in your clients' lives.

The reason as to *why* you're getting into the industry, will play an integral role in the path you choose to follow, your focus and your success. Knowing *why* you are getting into this profession, will also determine how hard you're willing to work and persevere through some of the many stressors and obstacles that you may encounter. Here are a few of them, based on my own experience.

As personal trainers, we have many additional daily stressors that can feel like a burden. For example, if you are an independent trainer you might have to travel from one location to your next session across a busy city. Do you get compensated for that travel time? Or you might have to juggle schedules at the last moment while still providing value to your clients. And, what if you're at (or hope to work at) a gym? Gyms have a lot of overhead and need to pay for expenditures, these are covered by taking a large percentage of a personal trainer's session rate. How do you train enough clients to cover for that percentage?

Clients also add a huge amount of extra stress to your life. For example, I've experienced the following situations: "One of my clients canceled today's session, which reduces my weekly wages. Am I able to get another client during this time?", "My client told me ten minutes before a session that she's traveling for two months. What can I do to make sure she stays healthy?", "My client told me 20 minutes before our session that they rolled their ankle last night, which completely changes their workout."

Another added difficulty is balancing your client's health with your own. Many trainers run from session to session, even within a gym, and take little time to care for themselves. With an unbalanced schedule, we deprioritize our health to care for others. Personal trainers will consistently have a lack of sleep, eat unhealthy food because we don't have enough time, or easily get sick because we're in contact with so many people.

Moreover, further stress can come from your relationship with your employer, your managers or employees, finding clients, and taking time to market yourself effectively. Knowing *why* you are a personal trainer will be a driving force that will keep you going through the difficult times.

And knowing your *why* will also keep you motivated to continue providing value to your clients. We know that physical fitness goes hand-in-hand with other parts of an individual's life, including their emotional, psychological, and spiritual needs. The personal trainer has a big part to play in balancing the daily lives of their clients. You, as a personal trainer, can bring so much value to your client's life through the fitness knowledge you coach, the motivation you provide, and the bond you share with them. Don't underestimate the difference that you can make in your clients' lives and the intrinsic value that you bring. You also have a special role to play in the community. You are a deliverer of motivation, deliverer of knowledge, an inspirer — you help people achieve their life goals.

We have looked at why finding the *why* is so important. Now we are going to look at how you can find that intrinsic motive.

Finding the deep motive as to *why* you want to be a personal trainer, can take time and some soul searching. But when you find the *why,* you will find yourself already beginning to focus on the aspects of personal training that are your passion.

If you don't know your motive, you can ask yourself some questions to direct your thinking. You can ask yourself, "What's my passion?" For example, do you enjoy coaching, mentoring and positively affecting lives. When you have a great session with a client, what was the highlight of that session? Was it seeing your client achieve a goal or was it connecting with your client on a new level that will enable you to help them? You can also ask yourself, "What are my goals?" For example, do you want to become an industry expert, to become the highest grossing trainer in Denver or to make a six-figure salary? What do you hope to get from this industry? For example, are you wanting increased knowledge in the profession, exposure as a personal trainer, or perhaps celebrity status?

I encourage you to take some time to think about what really inspires YOU want to become a personal trainer. When you know the answer to this question, or even a partial answer, you will be able to find your direction through this vast industry and your specific niche. Together we will be able to nurture that valuable intrinsic passion that you have to help people and find your purpose in the fitness industry.

Chapter Three

Facing Your Fears

"I learned that courage was not the absence of fear, but the triumph over it. The brave man is not he who does not feel afraid, but he who conquers that fear."
- Nelson Mandela-

Luke took the plunge and called Ted first thing in the morning. He was nervous, but he had reached a point of desperation, and that drove him to call. Ted was looking for an assistant personal trainer, but the role would be more demanding than the usual assistant position because Ted was needing someone to be actively involved in training his clients. It would be a step down for Luke, however, he would get a steady stream of clients and he would get the chance to work under direct supervision from Ted, a highly experienced and successful trainer and businessman.

"Hey, Luke, great to meet you," Ted was on crutches, but still managed to shake Luke's hand, "How are you doing today?"

Luke was surprised to note that despite the clichéd greeting, Ted was being completely sincere. He was genuinely interested in Luke and in his wellbeing. That was something that Luke would learn — Ted was authentic. He cared deeply about the people around him and did everything that he could to make sure his colleagues, friends, and clients were happy, healthy and achieved their goals. His gym was in the niche of health, wellness, and rehabilitation. He had partnered with a number of allied health professionals in the community, and they gave him a regular stream of clients that needed help. These clients ranged from those needing to lose weight to clients that had back injuries and were rehabilitating. Although the needs of the clients varied, they had one thing in common — they were all inspired by Ted's positive attitude and sincerity in caring for them.

Ted took Luke around the gym, it was small but looked professional. As they progressed through the different areas, Ted asked Luke about his background, his industry knowledge, and his career goals. He also questioned Luke as to *why* he became a personal trainer.

Luke smiled, "I've been thinking about that lately. I've asked myself quite a few questions about what inspires me and what I'm passionate about. I got down to the root — I genuinely want to help people. I've always been like that and when I see my clients progressing, I get a sense of accomplishment and fulfillment that money can't buy."

Ted saw a spark within Luke that resonated with his own values and passion for helping others.

"I've got a client now. Her name is Mary. She recently turned 80 and has been working with me for over a year. We have been working on losing weight and building strength and balance. When she first came here, she was using a Zimmer Frame. I have her file, I would like you to work with her today. Don't worry, everything is in here. Have a read through while I go chat with her," Ted hobbled out his office, into the studio. There was a spritely elderly lady warming up on the treadmill — with no Zimmer Frame and a smile on her face. Ted began to chat with her.

Luke had a look through the file. There were so many forms and records, even a referral letter from her physical therapist. Ted had compiled workout templates with notes on each workout that Mary had completed. He had recorded her progress, and it was amazing. This was like looking at a medical folder — it was so professional. Luke found the workout for the day, read through it and took a deep breath. He could do this...

"Hi Mary, my name is Luke. I'm going to be helping you today..."

Luke became engrossed in assisting Mary.

Ted watched Luke interact with Mary. He could see the passion and the enthusiasm, but he also noticed that there was much room for improvement in Luke's skills. He was a good personal trainer, good enough to compete with the other trainers out there, but with Ted's help, he could become excellent. He could become successful — possibly even more successful than Ted. Ted saw the potential in Luke, but he also saw the fears.

"Well done. That was a great session for Mary, I can see that she really took to you. I'd like to bring you on board. I think you will be a great asset to my clients, especially as I'm a bit limited in how I can assist them at the moment."

"Thanks, Ted, I really enjoyed working with her. The file was so comprehensive and professional. All those records and workout forms made it so easy to run the session," Luke was excited, he could learn so much from Ted. What an opportunity.

"Well, I see personal training as a profession. I see us as being the experts on health and wellness. The benefits and value that we can bring to people's lives are as beneficial as those in fields that we consider professional. If you bring value, you will be successful," Ted paused, "Building a personal training business is a bit like building a house. Before you can build a solid structure, you have to dig down deep to lay the foundation. It takes courage and hard work to go down deep enough, but without that — the building might stand for a short while — but it will collapse over time."

Luke nodded, "Well, foundations are important..."

"I'm actually talking about the 'digging down deep' part. When I first started considering opening a gym, I had quite a few fears that kept on surfacing — immobilizing me from going for it. I was afraid of going into debt, of wasting my time, and not being financially successful. I thought that I wasn't qualified enough, I was scared that I would mess-up my clients and be a failure. But then I started examining my fears. It took courage to sit down, dig deep and ask myself, 'What am I afraid of?' and then ask myself, 'If I failed completely, how could I repair my life?' Defining your fear prevents your brain from running away with concepts that can lead to paralyzed action. Fear will be there no matter what; we can choose to turn away from it or to confront it. So, Luke, I want to encourage you to ask yourself the difficult questions, 'Why am I not as successful as I want to be?', 'Why don't I have as many clients as I want to have?', 'What am I afraid of?'"

Luke would never have done this type of thing before, but he trusted Ted and he wanted to have what Ted had. Ted continued, "I want you to complete this Fear Setting exercise."

He handed Luke a sheet of paper. There was a table on it with four columns titled Fear, Define, Prevent and Repair.

"In the 'Fear' column you are going to define your fears. These answers will come from questioning *why* you have not been successful and *what* you fear. In the next column, 'Define,' you will define that fear, expand on it and be honest with yourself. Next to that in the 'Prevent' column you can write down ideas that could prevent your fears from coming to life, or at least decrease their likelihood. In the last column, 'Repair,' ask yourself what you could do to repair your life if the worst happened."

Luke nodded, he was nervous but knew that he had to dig deep if he wanted to lay the foundation to success. Ted held out his hand to shake Luke's, "One last thing, it was only when I stepped through those fears that I succeeded. I want you to do the same. Come back tomorrow and I'll have your contract ready."

Luke left feeling dazed. He couldn't believe all that had happened. For the first time in a long time, he could feel his passion for personal training beginning to return. He had a sense that life was going to change rapidly for the good. Luke felt hopeful.

***

> "The oldest and strongest emotion of mankind is fear, and the oldest and strongest kind of fear is fear of the unknown."
> - H.P. Lovecraft -

Many fitness enthusiasts get pushed away from achieving their purpose as personal trainers. What pushes them away? What *fears* do people have about following what they want to do? What do prospective personal trainers fear about the role? The answers to these questions differ for each person – some may lack the knowledge on how to create and grow their brand, and that fear prevents them from even trying. Others may wonder how they will create recognition of themselves in the fitness industry; they may feel that there are too many personal trainers out there to be successful, or there's not enough prospective clientele in their local geography. Many are aware of their gap in knowledge and skill and are scared of it. They don't think that they'll ever acquire the necessary knowledge and ability to be successful, and therefore they don't pursue their dreams.

Your personal fears may be leading to the following questions — Do I start on my own? Do I join a gym? Do I start at a school or university? Do I start with a sports team? Do I begin with group training? How do I hold a conversation with a stranger for a long period of time? How do I set my training price? Some fears are legitimate concerns and others are unfounded, yet they still demotivate us and can immobilize us — preventing us from pursuing our dreams.

FEAR SETTING EXERCISE

Let's change pace a little. We're launching straight into an exercise because the best way to learn something is to incorporate it into your life, immediately. This is an extremely important first exercise because it's going to force you to really think about your limitations. As you identify your fears or limiting beliefs, you'll realize that hidden in the fears are golden nuggets of positivity which you can take, expand, and work on, every day, every week, and every month until you're successful.

In this book, we're focusing on the professional and financial parts of your life, but I encourage you to go through this exercise, and the ones to follow, for all areas (your relationships, your emotional, psychological and spiritual aspects etc.).

Complete the exercise in the following order (example below):

Step 1. Take out a sheet of paper (or use your computer) and at the top of the page write "My Fears."

Step 2. Divide the page into four columns and title each of the rows as such (left to right) – Fear, Define, Prevent, Repair.

Step 3. In the left-hand column titled "Fear," write out the fears that you have. Ask yourself the difficult questions that begin with, "Why haven't I...?" and fill in the gap with the answers to those questions; the anxieties, frustrations, and activities you've put off.

For example, you may ask yourself the following questions:

Why haven't I started personal training yet?

Why haven't I obtained my first client?

Why haven't I achieved a full client schedule?

Why haven't I broken away from the gym I work at and gone out on my own even though I've wanted to for years?

Why haven't I opened my own fitness studio?

Why don't I have personal trainers working for me?

Why haven't I increased my per session rates?

Step 4. In the second column titled "Define," describe your fear as much as possible; take your time and be as specific as you can. This is a difficult activity and takes self-awareness.

Step 5. In the column titled "Prevent," write down ideas that could prevent your fears from coming to life, or at least decrease their likelihood.

Step 6. In the last column titled "Repair," describe what you could do to repair your life, or how you could ask for help if the worst case scenario happened.

Step 7. Take a deep breath and put the paper away until our next exercise.

Fear Setting Exercise Example:

	FEAR SETTING		
Fear	**Define**	**Prevent**	**Repair**
First job in a gym.	I'm not professionally ready, I don't have the motivation.	Get more experience, find a mentor.	Start in a different position (i.e. front desk attendant), expand my job search to other employer types (universities, sports teams, physical therapy clinics, etc.).
Open my first gym location.	Go into debt, waste my time, not be financially successful, I'm not professionally ready, I don't have the motivation, I don't have the finances.	Launch the gym with somebody (personal trainer, financier), find an advisor, crowdfunding.	Return to working as an employee, ask for financial help from friends/family.

By taking the time to complete the preceding exercise, you have already started to identify the things you fear and define the areas where you struggle, which most people don't take the time to consider. Defining fears allows you to discover elements of the unknown — areas and ideas that you didn't know about or if you were aware of those areas or issues, you ignored them and hoped they would solve themselves or disappear. When you leave your fears unchecked, it's easy for your brain to run away with the concepts and turn them into obstacles that seem impossible to overcome.

Congratulations on facing your fears. As we journey through this book, you will be stepping through each fear, or unknown element, and progressing towards success.

Chapter Four

Laying Your Foundation

"People with goals succeed because they know where they are going."
- Earl Nightingale -

"Fear will be there no matter what; we can choose to turn away from it or to confront it."

Ted's words rung in Luke's ears as he completed the Fear Setting Exercise that night. He found the courage to ask himself those difficult questions, and as he dug down deep into his thought processes, he found that he feared failing — and, therefore, indirectly feared and avoided many of the activities that would make him successful. He wanted to become an independent personal trainer and command a decent hourly rate. But what if he failed? How could he repair his life? Luke had been on the edge of failing; the edge of quitting. This opportunity to work with Ted was already a step in the right direction to putting the pieces back together and facing and conquering his fear.

"Morning Ted," Luke arrived early at the gym, Ted was already there preparing for the day. Ted got right down to business and gave Luke his contract and discussed Luke's Fear Setting Exercise. He was impressed.

"It takes a lot of courage to sit down and pinpoint one's fears. Well done. Many will walk away from that activity because, ironically, they are scared of it. But I've found that when I've had a good look at the 'giants of fear,' I've found them to be not so giant-like after all. I'm impressed at your level of commitment. I have more exercises for you to do. But first, we have a few clients to assist," Ted gave Luke a bunch of folders.

They were all neatly arranged and every one of them had the same collection of forms and documents that was in Mary's folder, just uniquely tailored to each client. Once more, Luke was inspired by Ted's care for his clients and the relationship that he built with each one.

The day passed by quickly and Luke loved every minute. He was more determined than ever to learn as much as possible. In the afternoon, Ted called Luke into his office.

"Remember I mentioned the exercises that I wanted you to complete? The following Commitment Exercises will help you figure out your short and long-term goals. They build on the Fear Setting Exercise that you completed last night." Ted passed Luke two forms. The first one was titled Partial Success Exercise and the second one was the Cost of Inaction Exercise.

Ted continued, "The Partial Success Exercise helps you to ask yourself what the benefits would be if you made an attempt at facing your fear (the ones you identified earlier). For example, someone might be scared of failing at their first job in a gym, but if they at least try, despite the fear, they would have built some skills and grown in confidence. As the saying goes, *you never know unless you try*," Ted continued, "The second exercise, The Cost of Inaction Exercise, gets you to take a look at the cost of *not* trying or *not* facing your fear. Once more, use your fears that you identified and ask yourself, 'If I avoid this fear for six months, one year and three years, how will it affect my life?' Think about the long-term effects of inaction on your professional life, your personal life, and even your family life."

Luke looked at the forms and felt a bit intimidated. It would be quite a mission to complete this. Ted smiled, he could totally relate to Luke's expression.

"This is part of the 'digging down deep' part before you lay the foundation. The deeper you dig, the firmer your foundation will be, Luke. The next part is laying the foundation — the beliefs, visions and motivations that are unseen but hold up and sustain one's life — and in your professional life... your business. Well, here's the first one. You've probably noticed the SMART goals for each client?" Luke nodded, he had been intrigued to see each client's goals meticulously recorded for each phase of their program. He had also been amazed at how many of them had actually achieved their goals with Ted's help.

"I live by a policy of *walk the talk*. I don't get my clients to complete any activity that I have not tried myself. You will be working closely with me, and I would like you to complete the SMART goals for your life. Go beyond just your profession, look at your personal life and even your family life. SMART goals enable you to break down a big dream into smaller more achievable pieces."

Ted then pointed to the wall behind him. Luke had noticed the collage of pictures relating to personal training and success. He also noticed a picture of a gym that looked very much like this one.

"That was my Vision Board before I stepped into owning a gym. I have a new one at home that I look at every day. I didn't want to throw this one away, so I put it here because it motivates me to continue to visualize success and embrace a winner's mentality. Creating this Vision Board, after completing all the exercises, helped me to define what I wanted out of life and helped me find my true calling... this," as he said that, Ted indicated towards his gym, "I would like you to create your own Vision Board over the next couple of days."

That evening, Luke sat down to start working on the various exercises. He had never done this sort of thing before, and a part of him felt that it was a waste of time. Then he remembered Ted's words to him as he was leaving, "Remember, in order to *achieve* something you've never done before, you must be willing to *become* somebody you've never been before." He was motivated to change.

***

> "Only I can change my life. No one can change it for me."
> - Carol Burnett -

It takes great courage to define and face your fears. In this section, we will build on the previous activity by looking a bit closer at your specific fears. We will also be completing two commitment exercises, which will help determine your goals in the short- and long-term. Once more, I encourage you to create milestones for every facet of your life.

EXTENSION OF THE FEAR SETTING EXERCISE

Partial Success Exercise

This activity is an extension of the Fear Setting Exercise, so please take out the exercise notes.

Complete the exercise in the following order (example below):

> **Step 1.** On a separate piece of paper, add the title "Benefits of an Attempt or Partial Success."

> **Step 2.** Under the title, write "Partial Success."

> **Step 3.** Create an equal amount of rows on this new page as you did with the Fear Setting Exercise (the rows are associated with the fears you noted).

> **Step 4.** For each fear, ask yourself what the benefits may be for partial success or an attempt.

For example: If your fear was... then an attempt or partial success would bring... benefits.

Benefits of an Attempt or Partial Success Example:

BENEFITS OF AN ATTEMPT/PARTIAL SUCCESS	
Fear	**Partial success**
First job in a gym.	Build skills, increase professional network, individuality, freedom, motivate me in the future.
Open my first gym location.	Build skills, build courage, individuality, freedom, motivate me in the future, increase financial success.

Cost of Inaction Exercise

The next exercise is also an extension of the Fear Setting Exercise, so please take out the exercise notes.

Complete the exercise in the following order (example below):

Step 1. On a separate piece of paper, add the title "Cost of Inaction."

Step 2. Divide the page into four columns and title each of the rows as such (left to right) 6-months, 1-year, 3-years, Rating (1–10).

Step 3. Create an equal amount of rows on this new page as you did with the Fear Setting Exercise (the rows are associated with the fears you noted).

Step 4. In the first three columns, ask yourself, "If I avoid this action for 6-months, 1-year, 3-years, how will it affect my life?" Think of the long-term effects of inaction on all aspects of your life including the emotional, spiritual, and physical areas.

Step 5. In the last column titled "Rating (1–10)," rate the cost of inaction for each fear, with 1 being the lowest and 10 being the highest cost.

Cost of Inaction Example:

COST OF INACTION			
6-months	**1-year**	**3-years**	**Rating (1 - 10)**
I'll feel like a coward.	I'll feel unfulfilled.	I'll feel unfulfilled, my opportunities are waning.	8
I'll feel unfulfilled.	I'm not living up to my life goals.	I've waited too long to fulfill my dreams, regret, shame.	9

COMMITMENT EXERCISES

S.M.A.R.T. Goals Exercise

The next exercise will be to set S.M.A.R.T. (Specific, Measurable, Action-oriented, Relevant, Time-bound) goals, used by many personal trainers during the client consultation. S.M.A.R.T. goals provide clearly outlined objectives and guidelines for success. They allow for big dreams to be broken down into smaller, more attainable actions.

Complete the exercise in the following order (example below):

Step 1. On a piece of paper write the title S.M.A.R.T. Goals and create six columns on the sheet with the following titles — Categories, Specific, Measurable, Action-oriented, Relevant, Time-bound.

Step 2. Under the "Categories" column write out all the areas where you want to establish goals. Although we are specifically focusing on your professional and financial goals, this activity will be beneficial for all aspects of your life.

Step 3. Under the "Specific" column, clearly define the goals you want to achieve.

Step 4. Under the "Measurable" column, clearly identify how you will measure each goal. How can you measure goal progress on a consistent basis?

Step 5. Under the "Action-oriented" column, outline specific milestones to attain the larger goal. What resources are necessary? How much effort will the goal take to achieve?

Step 6. Under the "Relevant" column, identify the personal reasons for chasing your goal. This column is the most important section. Having a real reason to achieve your goal, a driving passion, will provide added motivation to achieve the goal.

Step 7. Under the "Timeline" column, describe a clear and realistic deadline for your goals.

S.M.A.R.T. Goals Example:

		S.M.A.R.T. GOALS			
Cate-gories	**Speci-fic**	**Measur-able**	**Action-oriented**	**Rele-vant**	**Time-bound**
Profes-sional Goals.	I will be a full-time personal trainer at 24 Hour Fitness in Phoenix, Arizona.	Measured each day through client referral, and prospect acquisition.	Obtain one new client every four days, one new referral from each client after two training sessions, two new prospects each day, zero client loss.	I'm saving money to purchase a wedding ring for my girlfriend later this year.	Within five weeks.

Vision Board Exercise

The next exercise will be to create a Vision Board of your future successes. And I see some of your eyes rolling now, but this activity is extremely helpful.

Think about celebrity athletes, whether it's in American football, soccer, baseball, hockey, basketball, cricket or any other sport. From young adulthood through school, semi-professional and into elite status, athletes use vision boarding and other visualization techniques to help imagine positive outcomes. They envision what it's like to make the winning catch, what it's like to make the winning throw, to hit the winning home run, to score the winning goal, and to shoot the game-winning basket, because visualization primes the body and mind to accept the fact that we're winners. When you visualize success, your body and mind embrace a winner's mentality, which adopts the positive experience of achieving the goal. Athletes envision success on a daily, monthly, seasonal and yearly basis.

Visualization prepares you for success. Vision Boards create an additional sensory input to accept that you're going to be successful soon. We'll show you how to take your goals and create a vision board, so your goals become more than mantras. We'll guide you to collect images that express your goals, to make it easier for you to identify with a winning mentality.

Complete the exercise in the following order (example below):

> **Step 1.** Review all previous exercises (Fear Setting, Partial Success listing the Benefits of an Attempt or Partial Success, Cost of Inaction, S.M.A.R.T. Goals) and identify all the successful future outcomes your goals will provide you.
>
> For example, if you want to become a full-time personal trainer, a future outcome may be to own a house.
>
> **Step 2.** For each outcome, find an image (digital, physical) that identifies with the outcome.

Step 3. Place all images on a board or sheet of paper.

Step 4. Visit your vision board on daily basis to inspire your future success, today.

Vision Board Example:

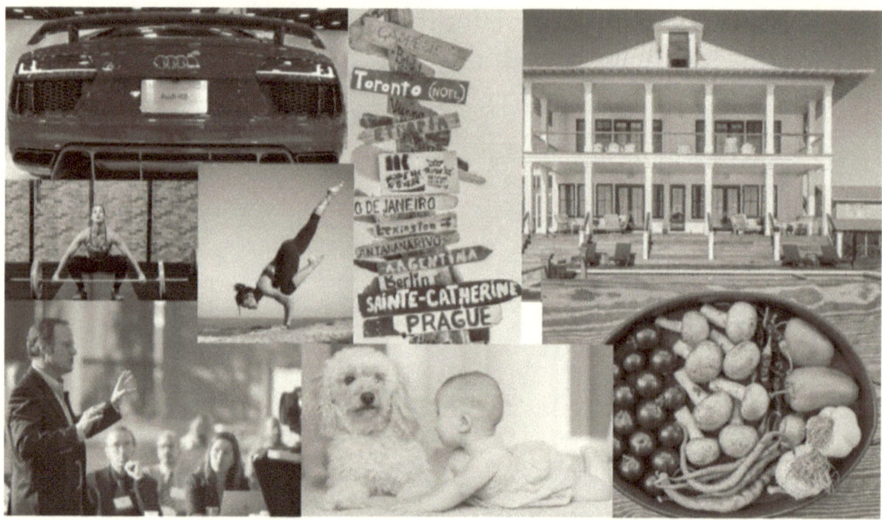

The ideas and activities so far are different from what you've been doing. Different and better whether you're a prospective personal trainer or an experienced personal trainer with a full schedule. You're reading this book because there are stressors in your life that you can't shake off or goals that you're not hitting as a personal trainer. If you're already skipping over the previous exercises, rolling your eyes, or thinking that this book isn't for you, ask yourself, *"Why?"* Have you tried these exercises before? If you have, have you stuck to your success roadmap?

And if you haven't tried the exercises before, tell yourself the following:

> "In order to achieve something you've never done before, you must be willing to become somebody you've never been before."
> - source unknown-

As you journey through this book and towards success, the path will feel uncertain and uncomfortable. But why uncertain and uncomfortable? To create this new success in your life — to hit the ground running as a first-time personal trainer, to increase your price per session, to create a passive income — you must do something you've never done before. You'll feel uncomfortable because you're trying new activities. You'll feel uncertain because it's hard to give up the comfort of your current, known situation.

When I started trying these techniques, I felt uncertain, uncomfortable, and scared. It was scary to move away from industry norms and my personal training coworkers because I was comfortable. My finances, at the time, were working for me. But I didn't want my finances to just be "working" for me. I wanted more. I needed more. I wanted to succeed. I wanted to live a life of abundance while still working as a personal trainer.

This deep desire for more, caused me to persevere in applying the techniques mentioned throughout this book. I found that defining my fears, goals and career path in detail helped set me on my path to success. I experienced more focus, determination and passion. It really helped that I was able to define what was holding me back, plan how to work effectively, and help more people along the way. I created financial freedom, new daily enthusiasm and energy in my clients because they could feel my positive change. The activities and ideas described here helped bring me into areas I never dreamed of such as creating fitness products, creating an independent personal training business and writing a health blog.

In the next part of this book, we will be laying the path that will shorten your window to becoming a successful, experienced personal trainer. You will find all the tools, the exercises, and the systems to push you towards success — no matter the level of your experience.

Chapter Five

Your Tools

"Accept yourself, your strengths, your weaknesses, your truths,
and know what tools you have to fulfill your purpose."
- Steve Maraboli –

It was late afternoon, the last client, Peter, had just left. Luke and Ted had spent the last 15 minutes of the session going over Peter's diet and his goals for the next week. Peter had come to Ted over a month ago to help him change his lifestyle. He was heavily overweight and shuffled instead of walked. His daughter was getting married in a year's time and Peter wanted to walk her down the aisle without feeling out of breath and embarrassed. They had gradually changed his diet. Peter's lifestyle needed a big change, but trying to change everything would have caused him to feel overwhelmed and quit. So Ted had encouraged him to set small goals, and they were slowly tackling the changes step-by-step. The results spoke for themselves, Peter was steadily losing weight and improving his fitness, and he felt confident he would reach his goals. In the last few minutes, they had spoken about courage — the courage to change and the courage to persevere.

As they headed into Ted's office, Ted said, "Luke, you've shown tremendous courage over the last week. I have seen you work through some of your own fears, you've asked yourself the difficult questions and made a plan to step through those fears. I've also seen you take what you learned and have already been applying it to how you work with the clients. I think you are ready for the next step."

Luke felt excited. It had been a difficult, yet amazing, week.

After writing down his goals and creating his Vision Board, he felt grounded and focused. He also felt as if he was starting from the beginning and learning how to be a personal trainer for the first time.

"You've already worked with the client files quite a bit. Here are the templates to those files. You'll find the Client Intake Forms, Medical Release Forms and Physical Assessment Forms in this file," He gave Luke a bundle of documents in a file and carried on, "I'd like you to learn these like the back of your hand. Also, here are the templates for the exercise programs and meals."

"I noticed that you had all the forms, but I didn't realize that you worked from templates for the exercise aspect and the meals. Why do you do that?" Luke was genuinely interested. He had prided himself in being able to draw up a program and meal plan from scratch for each client even though it took a lot of time and effort.

"Well, once I had worked for a couple of years, I realized that I was actually using a mental pattern or routine whenever I had clients that had similar needs. It dawned on me that I would save a tremendous amount of time if I just drew up templates and used them instead of starting from scratch," Ted smiled.

"So, do you fit the client into the template?"

"Absolutely not! We adapt the template to the client. Each client is different, and each client is on a journey and will change on a weekly and yearly basis. What works for a client today, will not work in the future. This is the reason why we don't just use templates and fit our clients into them, but we start with a template, like the bones of a skeleton, and build and update them with client-specific information. As the client journeys through their goals, we update and adapt the program."

Luke nodded, "That makes sense. It simplifies things a lot and I guess you can focus more on the client and their needs than coming up with a whole new program."

"Exactly, and it gives you more time for the other aspects of your business. Which leads me to the next point. You *are* your business and you need tools to run your business. So many personal trainers start working without knowing how to run a business. Sales and marketing are more of an afterthought, and the administrative tasks of running a business tend to be neglected. So, here are some of the forms that I would like you to look at and learn how to complete," Ted gave Luke a folder marked Business Documents. Inside the file, he found various materials for running a business, such as insurance forms, release of liability forms for the client, and payment templates. He had never worked with this side of a business before, but he was willing to learn.

"Ted, you mentioned sales and marketing. Surely we don't need to market ourselves? I've always just presented myself and my services to clients. I haven't really worked on sales and marketing." Luke was actually weak at sales and marketing. He didn't really know how to sell or market himself and was reluctant to even attempt it.

"You know, I used to think that too until I read various books on business, sales, and marketing. I found my niche and my passion, and I realized that if I wanted to grow as a business and bring value to my clients, I *had* to market myself. Here are a few sales and marketing materials. Have a look at them and think about how you would market yourself. How would you ask for a sale? How can you take the services that you offer and share them with your community?"

Inside that folder marked Sales and Marketing, Luke found drafts of Ted's company logo, business cards, flyers and price sheets. He also found a few notes on the various books that Ted had read and used.

As Luke traveled home, he reflected on all he had learned that day. The folders were heavy in his bag, and a part of him felt overwhelmed at all the tasks that Ted had given him to complete. However, working with Ted and his clients had taught him one thing — small goals, completing tasks step-by-step and perseverance. He thought of Peter and the challenge that he was facing head-on with Ted's help... it was inspiring. If Peter could find the courage to change and slowly work on overcoming his obstacles, so could Luke find the courage to tackle each task one step at a time.

***

> "The journey matters as much as the goal."
> -Kalpana Chawla-

In our journey so far, we have already identified the issues with the industry, the issues with becoming a personal trainer, and the issues holding a personal trainer back from success. You've looked inside yourself, recognized fears, sought limiting beliefs, and identified anxieties that have held you back so far. The first part of the book was the hardest emotionally, but essential in building a solid foundation that will enable you to be successful in the short term and the long term. In this section, we'll present the tools to help you succeed.

Some of these materials will speak more to specific types of trainers, such as gym owners and independent contractors because they need to be successful at large-scale sales, marketing, and business operations. However, I strongly urge you to read each section as there are helpful tips in each part and although you may not need all the information right now, you may need it in the future. It may inspire you to open your own gym or become an independent personal trainer.

The materials outlined below are designed to provide value to your clients, your business, and ultimately to you.

> Value is the catalyst to success

Value works as a catalyst to success – the more value you

provide your clients, the more value they return to you, the more value you feel in yourself, the more value you provide your clients, and on and on.

In this section, I'll discuss examples of forms, questionnaires, templates, assessments, and other materials. Find the full versions of these documents on my website here: www.MakeMoneyPersonalTraining.com

PERSONAL TRAINING MATERIALS

To begin, let's take a look at personal training materials – the activities and information that will provide a basis while you're meeting with clients. This will be most helpful for newer personal trainers though experienced trainers may find additional tips to update their frameworks.

Search online for personal training material and you'll be flooded with information. What are some of the basic personal training materials you need to be comfortable with? Here's a list of training materials that you need to understand:

- Client Intake Forms
- Medical Release Form
- Physical Assessment Form
- Food Journal
- Exercise Program Templates
- Meal Templates
- Client Session Sign-in Sheet

Let me answer one of your first questions immediately. Nutrition and exercise program templates? It's much easier and quicker to build and customize workouts if you work from a template. Personal trainers use templates all the time. These can be actual templates taken from a book or an online source that we copy and adapt, or they can be mental frameworks that we form based on years of experience. To the experienced trainer who has worked with many clients, it becomes second nature to use those mental frameworks (aka templates) to assess new clients and to design exercise and nutrition programs based on their understanding of the client's unique abilities, needs, and goals.

It is quicker to use a template as a foundation from which to build a program than to start from scratch with each new client. You have a template, and you mix and match exercises based on the client's goals and assessments. By using templates, you can literally save hundreds of hours each year on program creation.

Not only will it save you time, but your programs will be more effective because you can focus on customizing and adapting the program specifically for each client. Each client is different, and each client is on a journey and will change on a weekly and yearly basis. What works for a client today, will not work in the future. This is the reason why we don't just use templates and fit our clients into them, but we start with a template, like the bones of a skeleton, and build and update them with client-specific information. Adopt the proven path, simplify your methods, and use templates.

To save you time, I'll give you the templates: the frameworks that will help you effectively create training programs for your clients where you can easily replace the exercises depending on the individual goals of your client.

Successful personal trainers take opportunities to simplify and save time (and money!) whenever possible. Let's dive in!

Client Intake Forms

Client Intake Forms are a bundle of documents that your prospects and clients need to fill out. The Client Intake Forms I'm referring to are the Par-Q, Activity History, Nutrition History, Attitude Questionnaire, Goal Setting, and anything else you deem important. My Client Intake Forms are one bundle, however, I've known many personal trainers that separate the material into distinct documents. Choose whichever option suit you.

Moreover, these forms will take 30–60 minutes to review with your prospect and it's important you do NOT skip over this step. This is your first opportunity to gain insight, look professional, and deliver value to your future client.

The **PAR-Q**, or Physical Activity Readiness Questionnaire, is used as a short screening for people about to begin an exercise program. This document should be completed first as it can identify any contraindications (reasons why the client cannot participate) to specific exercises or an exercise program. The PAR-Q has the following content:

- Client name
- Client contact information
- Emergency contact information
- Physician contact information
- Questions related to high-risk factors, such as, "Do you feel pain in your chest when you are performing physical exercise?"
- Questions related to present and past health history, such as, "Do you have low blood pressure?"
- Questions related to family health history, such as, "Have any of your relatives had a premature death before age 50?"

PAR-Q Example:

PAR-Q-FORM

All information received on this form will be treated as strictly confidential.

Please fill out the forms **completely and accurately.**

Date: _____________________   Name: _______________________

Date of birth: ___________________   Sex: _______

Weight (if known): ____________   Height (if known): ____________

Address: ____ Street

_____________________ City _____________ State ____________ Zip

Phone (H): ____________________   (W): ____________________

E-mail address: ____________________

Emergency contact information

Name: ____________________   Relationship: _______________

Phone (H): ____________________   (W): ____________________

Personal physician

Name: ____________________

Phone (H): ____________________   Fax: ____________________

For the complete document, visit MakeMoneyPersonalTraining.com

The **Activity History Form** is used as an overview of a person's physical activity on a daily basis. The information collected here will help you identify areas of opportunity, or value, to help your client. The Activity History Form asks questions such as:

- Client occupation
- Stress levels
- Basic exercise ability, such as, "Can you currently walk 4 miles briskly without fatigue?"
- Current exercise frequency
- Current fitness routine, exercises, difficulty level

Activity History Form Example:

ACTIVITY HISTORY

All information received on this form will be treated as strictly confidential.

Please fill out the forms **completely and accurately.**

Are you presently employed?　☐ Yes　☐ No

What is your present occupational position? _______________________________

Name of Company: _______________________________

Does your current job require travel?　☐ Yes　☐ No

On a scale of 1-10, how would you rate your stress level (1=very low 10=very high)? _____

List your 3 biggest sources of stress:

a. _________________　b. _________________　c._________________

Date of your last physical examination performed by a physician: _________________

How often do you currently participate in an exercise program?

☐ Never　　☐ 1-2 time/week　　☐ 3-4 times/week　　☐ 5-7 times/week

For the complete document, visit MakeMoneyPersonalTraining.com

The **Nutrition Overview Form** is used as an indication of a person's nutrition on a daily basis. The information collected here will help you identify areas of opportunity, or value, to help your client. The Nutrition Overview Form reviews the following content:

- Client's energy levels
- Calories consumed
- Caffeine intake
- Vitamin and supplement intake
- Smoking intake
- Water intake
- Sugar intake
- If the client follows a specific diet plan

Nutrition Overview Form Example:

NUTRITION OVERVIEW

All information received on this form will be treated as strictly confidential.
Please fill out the forms **completely and accurately.**

Do you feel drops in your energy levels throughout the day?   Yes   No

Do you know how many calories you eat per day?   Yes How many? _______   No

How many cups of coffee do you drink per day? ____________

How many glasses of alcohol do you consume per day? ___________

Do you take vitamins or supplements?   Yes   No

If yes, please explain below: ____

____

Do you smoke?   Yes   Amount per day _____ Since what age _____   No

Do you follow any specific dietary intake plan?   Yes   No

If yes, please explain below: ____

____

In general, how do you feel about you nutritional habits?: ____________________________

The **Attitude Questionnaire** is used to gain insight into your client's psychology around exercise and their physical abilities. The information collected here will help you identify how to best motivate and sell to your client. The Attitude Questionnaire reviews the following content:

- Client's feelings around physical exercise
- Perception of their current fitness abilities, such as, "Rate your present flexibility"
- Ability to stick to an exercise program

Attitude Questionnaire Example:

ATTITUDE QUESTIONNAIRE

All information received on this form will be treated as strictly confidential.

Please fill out the forms **completely and accurately.**

Do you have any negative feeling towards, or have you had any bad experience with, physical activity programs?

Yes ☐ *No* ☐

If yes, please explain below: ___________________________________

Do you have any negative feeling towards, or have you had any bad experience with, fitness training and evaluation?

Yes ☐ *No* ☐

If yes, please explain below: ___________________________________

Do you often start exercise programs but then find yourself unable to stick with them?

Yes ☐ *No* ☐

How much time are you willing to devote to an exercise program? ___*days/week* ___*minutes/day*

Can you exercise during your work day? ☐ *Yes* ☐ *No*

Would an exercise program benefits your job? ☐ *Yes* ☐ *No*

The **Goal Setting Form** is used as an overview of your client's goals – get as specific as possible. The information collected here will help you identify how to best motivate and sell to your client. The Goal Setting Form has the following content:

- Purpose of an exercise and nutrition program
- S.M.A.R.T. health goals – identical to the S.M.A.R.T. goal exercise you did earlier in this book
- Expectations of a personal trainer

Goal Setting Form Example:

GOAL SETTING

All information received on this form will be treated as strictly confidential.

Please fill out the forms **completely and accurately.**

To increase your chances of success at achieving your goals, its best to use the S.M.A.R.T. goal system (Specific, Measurable, Attainable, **RELEVANT**, and Time-based). Example below.

Specific	Measurable	Attainable	Relevant	Time-based
I will walk 15,000 steps every week day for the next three months	Smart phone or step counter	I already walk 10,000 steps every week day, so a 5,000 step increase is manageable	To increase my heart health because I have a family history of heart disease	Every week day for the next 3 months

Please define your health goals using the S.M.A.R.T. system.

GOAL ONE:: ____

GOAL TWO:: ____

GOAL THREE:: ____

For the complete document, visit MakeMoneyPersonalTraining.com

Medical Release Form

The **Medical Release Form** is used to receive clearance from a client's physician. It's good practice to have any client who answered "Yes" to questions in the PAR-Q High Risk section to get medical clearance and may be good practice to request all clients have their physicians complete the form. The Medical Release Form has the following content:

- Recent physical examination confirmation
- Pre-existing medical conditions
- Medication(s) that can affect exercise
- Optional physician recommendations

Physical Assessment Form

The **Physical Assessment Form** consists of a series of activities to test the physical abilities of your prospects and clients. The first time you test a prospect, the assessment will take 30–60 minutes. Take your time and pay attention to how your prospect moves and how they feel while performing each assessment.

The assessment is a short series of tests, but in all honesty, you consistently test your clients. To gain a full picture of your client's physical abilities, it may take two to ten training sessions before you understand your client's capabilities. The more attention that you pay to your clients, the faster you can create an appropriate program, and the faster you can deliver value.

It's good practice to perform the Physical Assessment periodically (eg. every six months) to provide consistent feedback to each client. No need to worry if you don't have access to the equipment necessary for the following activities. Your client may know the information or you can find other tests that use the equipment you do have. Additionally, there are dozens more tests that can be performed in this section; I'm providing the tests that have worked for me.

The Physical Assessment Form has the following content:

- Basic physical measurements – height, weight, heart rate, blood pressure
- Body composition/body fat test
- Static postural assessment – tests a client's posture, which gives insight into their daily stressors, body tightness, muscle weakness, and effects of previous injury
- Stork stand balance test – tests a client's balance. If a client cannot stand without losing balance, you need to have their physician fill out a Medical Release Form before they continue with the Physical Assessment and exercise
- Comprehensive movement assessment – deep squat, inline lunge, shoulder mobility, active straight-leg raise
- Endurance assessment – there are many endurance assessments and I use the Balke treadmill test

Physical Assessment Form Example:

Physical Fitness Assessment

Name: _____________________ Date: _____________________

Heart Rate: Resting heart rate: _____________________ bpm

Blood Pressure: Resting blood pressure: _________/____________ mmHg

BODY COMPOSITION ASSESSMENT

BMI Calculator

Weight (lb.): _____________________ Height (in.): _____________________

If necessary, convert to metric units using the following:

Weight (lbs.) x 0.454 = Weight in kilograms (kg)

Height (in.) x 0.0254 = Height in meters (m)

Weight (kg): _____________________ Height (in.): _____________________

Calculate BMI: Weight (kg) / Height^2 (m)

BMI: _____________________

Note: *Refer to BMI visual aids for results*

For the complete document, visit MakeMoneyPersonalTraining.com

Food Journal

The **Food Journal** is used to assess the current state of your client's nutrition, to make them aware of what they're putting into their body, and allows you to both be fully aware of the client's commitment to their goals. All of these reasons add value to your services. The Food Journal shows you really care about your clients – you care about what they eat, what they drink, and even what they feel about food.

Most personal trainers who use a Food Journal will ask their clients to record their meals for three days, including one weekend day. I ask my clients to report on seven days so we can both have a complete understanding of their nutrition. The Food Journal has the following content:

- Weekly or daily calendar
- Breakdown of nutrient types (i.e. carbohydrates) *or* meals (i.e. breakfast)
- Water intake
- Emotions around each meal (strongly recommended) – understanding how people feel about their meals and why they eat, can help minimize clients' bad eating habits. For example, if a client drinks coffee at 9 a.m., eats sweets at 2 p.m. and then feels sluggish and angry around 3 p.m., you can assimilate these negative feelings to poor food choices
- General daily activity (optional) – allows for a full picture of a person's chosen daily health activities on one sheet
- Sleep gauge (optional) – sleep affects hunger and taking note of sleep allows for a full picture of a person's daily health activities

Exercise program templates

The **Weight Loss Exercise Template** is an exercise program used for clients who want to lose weight. Clients will undergo a mixture of strength and endurance training. The Weight Loss Exercise Template has the following characteristics:

- 2 – 3 sets
- 10 – 20 repetitions (reps)
- Light weight
- Low – moderate intensity
- Full body daily workouts
- Frequent rest days

The **Strength Gain Exercise Template** is an exercise program used for clients who want to gain strength. Clients will undergo a mixture of strength training and HIIT (High Intensity Interval Training) exercises (*Note*: HIIT can be replaced with endurance exercises). The Strength Gain Exercise Template has the following characteristics:

- 4 sets
- 5 – 8 reps (with most exercises)
- Moderate – heavy weight
- Daily routines are separated into "splits" or programs. The most popular strength splits workout the following muscle groups (split into different workout days) – Chest/abs, back/calves, shoulders/abs, legs, upper body/abs
- Endurance or HIIT workouts 2 – 3 days a week

The **Heart Health Exercise Template** is an exercise program used for clients who want to strengthen their heart and increase energy. Clients will undergo a mixture of light strength training and frequent endurance workouts. The Heart Health Exercise Template has the following characteristics:

- 2 - 3 sets
- 10 – 20 reps
- Light weight
- Low – moderate intensity
- Full body daily workouts
- Frequent endurance workouts

The **Athletic Exercise Template** is an exercise program used for clients who want to increase their athletic ability. Client's will undergo a mixture of weight amounts and exercise types. The Athletic Exercise Template has the following characteristics:

- Mixture of weight intensities – light, moderate, heavy
- Mixture of exercise types – power, strength, endurance
- 5 – 10 reps
- Full body daily workouts
- Frequent rest
- Workout programs will change based on in- or out-of-season sports

The **Balanced Exercise Template** is an exercise program used for clients who want to have a balanced body. Clients will undergo a mixture of strength and endurance training. The Balanced Exercise Template has the following characteristics:

- Light – moderate weight
- Power and strength exercises
- 8 – 12 reps
- 2 – 3 sets
- Focus on creating bi-lateral (both sides) muscular strength balance
- Focus on strengthening the 7 primal movement patterns – squat, lunge, push, pull, twist, bend, gait (i.e. walking, jogging, sprinting)

Meal Templates

The **Weight Gain Meal Template** is used for clients who want to gain weight. The Weight Gain Meal Template has the following characteristics:

- Multiple meals
- A high amount of calories
- A high amount of protein and carbohydrates

The **Low Carb Meal Template** is used for clients who want to avoid high amounts of carbohydrates. The Low Carb Meal Template has the following benefits:

- Reverses type 2 diabetes and metabolic syndrome
- Reduces sugar intake and encourages weight loss
- Reduces heartburn and calms the stomach
- Normalizes blood pressure

The **Gluten-free Meal Template** is used for clients who want to avoid gluten. The Gluten-free Meal Template has the following characteristics:

- Improves the quality of life for people with celiac disease or gluten sensitivity
- Improves cholesterol levels, promotes digestive health, increases energy

The **Paleo Meal Template** is used for clients who want to emulate our hunter-gatherer ancestors. The Paleo Meal Template has the following benefits:

- Low in sodium, high in potassium, high in fiber, high in antioxidant vitamins, high in minerals, high in "good" fats
- Lowers cholesterol, increases metabolism
- Reduces the risk of high blood pressure, strokes, and certain cancers

The **Vegan Meal Template** is used for clients who want to avoid food products made from animals. The Vegan Meal Template has the following benefits:

- Decreases weight, blood sugar levels, Type 2 diabetes
- Lowers cancer risk, arthritis, Alzheimer's disease, kidney dysfunction

The **Mediterranean Meal Template** is used for clients who want a diet consistent with those around the Mediterranean Sea (i.e. Spain, France, Italy, Greece, Turkey, Morocco). The Mediterranean Meal Template has the following benefits:

- Lowers blood pressure, heart attacks, obesity, type 2 diabetes, premature death, cancer risk, Parkinson's disease, Alzheimer's disease, strokes
- Lowers "bad" cholesterol levels, encourages weight loss

Client Session Sign-in Sheet

If you work for a gym, the clients usually sign-in at the front desk, providing a written record of attendance (signed by the client). I've known many personal trainers who did not have a sign-in sheet in place and the client didn't pay for the sessions at the end of the month when the invoice was due. Client session sign-in sheets help inspire clients to pay their bills because there's a signed log of attendance. In addition, a client session sign-in sheet establishes your professionalism and creates a respectful business.

ESSENTIAL PIECES OF EQUIPMENT

Understanding the essentials of personal training equipment is important for success. What are some exercise tools that will make you more successful during a training session? Below, I outline Basic, Intermediate and Advanced equipment to help you succeed.

Basic Equipment

- Self-myofascial release tools (i.e. tennis ball, lacrosse ball) – tools to help release tension in the muscle and fascial tissue (the tissue that holds your body together)
- Jump rope – not for all clients, but it's highly effective for those clients that can use it. Additionally, it's lightweight, affordable, and can fold into any sized bag.

Intermediate Equipment

- Weights
- Yoga mat
- Kettlebells
- Weight vest
- Resistance bands
- TRX Suspension Training

Advanced Equipment

- Sports-specific equipment such as boxing equipment, overspeed training
- Battle rope
- Ladder
- Athletic cones

Additionally, there are non-exercise materials you should have nearby during a session. These are outlined below.

Basic Materials

- Notebook
- Pens
- Client session sign-in sheet
- Clipboard – to take notes throughout the session on the exercise and nutrition plans

- Water and a small towel
- Mobile phone – to reach your next clients and follow up with fitness and nutrition advice
- Exercise and nutrition plans – to consistently update with your client's feedback

Intermediate Materials

- First aid kit
- Spare clothing – if you're a personal trainer, you'll understand why you need a change of clothes. You're moving around a lot during your training sessions and you may even get a little dirty. Additionally, personal trainers have to balance their schedules with their own fitness programs, many times not having enough time to shower before their next client session. An additional change of clothes helps the personal trainer stay professional and comfortable
- Sunscreen – depending on geographic location and training type
- Deodorant
- Chalk – used for outdoor training, being creative such as drawing a ladder on the ground. Chalk can save time and money
- Watch or timer – it can look more professional to use a device other than your smartphone to track time during a training session, so using a watch or timer is good practice
- Flexible tape measure – used for measuring client body measurements during the initial fitness consultations, and periodically to measure milestones and goal attainment

Advanced (go the extra mile) Materials

- Kleenex – establishes comfort in a training session by thinking ahead
- Hair ties – for those clients who have long hair. When clients are moving around and sweating, long hair can be a nuisance. It's good practice to think ahead about the comfort of your clients

Recommended Personal Training Books

To continue your own education, you can read books, journals, and attend events and seminars that are interesting. Some of the best personal training books (depending on your niche) that I've found are:

- *Advances in Functional Training* by Michael Boyle
- *Essentials of Strength Training and Conditioning* (NSCA book)
- *Athletic Body in Balance* by Gray Cook
- *Movement – The Functional Movement System (FMS)* by Gray Cook
- *How to Eat, Move and Be Healthy* by Paul Chek
- *Biochemical Individuality – The key to understanding what shapes your health* by Roger J. Williams
- *Gait Analysis – Normal and Pathological Function* by Jacquelin Perry (if you enjoy biomechanics)

There are thousands more fitness books out there with great information. Find your niche, find your passion and dive into the topics.

Note: I don't have any partnerships with the aforementioned books. Please refer to the Recommended Reading section for more details on the listed titles.

BUSINESS MATERIALS

For those personal trainers who are not employees, you need to become familiar with the business tools that will make you successful. We'll go over the necessary business forms you need to create success as an independent trainer and gym owner. These materials are completely necessary to be a successful personal trainer.

- Insurance – General Liability, Disability, Professional Liability

- Release of Liability Form
- Payment Templates - Direct Debit and Invoice

Insurance Materials

Insurance is necessary for all personal trainers:

General Liability insurance protects you if you're sued by a client due to injuries (trip and fall incident) or damages. This insurance is recommended for all trainers.

Disability insurance protects you in case you are injured and it helps pay your bills even when you are not working. This insurance is recommended for all trainers.

Professional Liability insurance protects against professional negligence or failure to perform as a competent professional. If you have a business partner or employ personal trainers, professional liability insurance is highly recommended.

The **Release of Liability Form** is a legal document between you and your client that addresses the possibility of an accident occurring and is a standard contract used throughout the fitness industry. Many clients will sign this document without reading it, which is not helpful to anyone. It's good practice to input sections that require your clients to acknowledge a statement with their initials or signature, adding additional focus to the document.

Payment Forms

The **Direct Debit Form** requests your clients' banking information so that you can automatically withdraw money from their account on a regular basis. This form requires much security and assumption of risk on your part, but it makes it much easier for you and your client to work together.

The **Invoice** is a bill that breaks down your services and cost, and is delivered to your client at the time of payment.

SALES AND MARKETING MATERIAL

Sales and marketing materials are needed by all personal trainers though some materials will be more valuable than others. For example, personal trainers who work for a gym may not need to create their own prospect lists, but they will still need a website. Even if you work at a gym where they provide most of the materials for you, you can and should have your own. What sales and marketing material will help make you successful? Here's a list to get us started:

- Company Logo
- Business Card
- Flyer
- Price Sheet
- Prospect List
- Client Referral Form
- Website(s)
- Social Media Content Bundle

A **Company Logo** is a visual representation of your brand. For prospects who haven't met you yet, it's the first object of yours they'll encounter. A logo has many benefits, including the following:

- Provides you with an individual identity (aka brand)
- Differentiates you from other personal trainers
- Makes you stand out in the fitness industry
- Shows commitment to your business
- Attracts more clients
- Shows professionalism
- Makes you memorable
- Adds a visual identity to accompany your business name

Business Cards may seem unnecessary in today's modern world where many aspects of life are going digital, but the business card will not be replaced anytime soon. Business cards have the following benefits:

- Most effective direct marketing tool
- It's the first impression of your brand
- Provides a continuous physical representation of your brand that the prospect can refer to
- Shows you're prepared at any time
- Convenient and quick contact source
- Provides credibility
- Provides a personal touch to exchanging contact information

A **Flyer**, like the business card, may seem unnecessary because of our digital age, but they are also not going away anytime soon. A flyer has your logo, company name, services and may even have pricing information. Flyers provide many benefits for your business including:

- An effective direct marketing tool
- Feedback from prospects because you get to see how many flyers are taken up at a location
- Affordable, visual marketing tool
- Simple and easily read advertisement

A **Price Sheet** is a written representation of your services and prices. There are many ways to price your services (more in the Pricing section later on). The following are the benefits of a Price Sheet:

- Visual aid, providing immediate value to prospects
- Inspires credibility
- Shows professionalism
- Enhances discount pricing (if used)

A **Prospect List** is the most important aspect of selling your services. Without a prospect, there is no sale. Employees trade some of their paycheck for access to a prospect list (amongst other things), whereas independent personal trainers and gym owners need to create their own lists. How do you create this list? Here are a few suggestions:

- Partner with somebody who has complementary (similar, but not overlapping) services so they can refer prospects to you, such as with wellness coaches, doctors and physical therapists, nutritionists, other specialty gyms (i.e. yoga), healthy restaurants, and local sports apparel stores
- Host an event
- Partner with or attend an event
- Referrals (family, friends, coworkers, clients)
- Digital marketing (website, social media, advertising)
- Write a blog or write a post for an established blog
- Direct mailers (flyers) targeted at your niche market
- Join an online personal training program

A **Client Referral Form** is a way to capture referrals from prospects and clients. Just like with sales, if you don't ask for the referral, you're probably not going to get it. Referrals provide the following benefits:

- Generates leads
- Improves conversion rate (selling your services) because the new prospect trusts the person who referred them
- Reduces your marketing costs
- Improves client accountability because they know another client in your community
- Increases client engagement
- Referrals lead to more referrals

A business **Website** today is like having a business card 50 years ago — it's smart and expected for any modern business. There's no need to have a flashy and expensive website, but also avoid creating an ugly site. Simplicity is fine and affordable. A website can provide the following benefits:

- More people who come into contact with you (physically or digitally) means more potential sales — period
- Increase the number of people who come in contact with your brand
- Access to you and information on your services
- Easily expand into additional avenues, such as selling products, writing a blog, and partnerships
- Extends your local reach
- Shows credibility
- Simple way to advertise and build your brand
- Improves customer service
- Less expensive than traditional marketing

A **Social Media Content Bundle** is a pack of content templates that make it easier for you to post on social media. It provides a framework to simply upload the content you write into an easily digestible social media format, whether that's Facebook, LinkedIn, Twitter, Snapchat, YouTube, and more. Social media marketing provides the following benefits:

- More contact = more sales
- Increased conversion (turning a prospect into a client) rates
- Increases the number of people who come in contact with your brand (aka increases inbound traffic)
- Decreases marketing costs because the templates save time spent organizing posts
- Increased brand recognition
- Increased brand loyalty
- Increases your authority (expertise)
- Increases your reach and client experience

To use the Social Media Content Bundle, you need to first set up your social media accounts. I highly recommend creating a business account for each social media outlet you're using instead of combining personal and business accounts on the same social media account.

Appropriate attire

Easily overlooked but an essential aspect of promoting your brand and building a reputation is being a professional — successful personal trainers dress the part. Personal training professional attire looks like this:

1. Branded t-shirt – if you work for a gym, they will most likely give you a branded t-shirt or top. If you're an independent trainer or if you work for a gym and you're exercising, wear branded clothing that has your business name, personal name, phone number, email address or website. All of this information is helpful so the prospect can contact you even if they don't meet you in person.
2. Exercise clothing – dress the part. Being successful at marketing means creating your individual brand, which begins with how you dress. If you don't look like a personal trainer, your prospect pool will diminish.
3. Athletic shoes – aim for comfort, because you'll be standing for hours each day.

Appropriate brand presentation

> "All of us need to understand the importance of branding. We are CEOs of our own companies: Me Inc. To be in business today, our most important job is to be head marketer for the brand called You."
> –Tom Peters–

Your brand is a presentation of your philosophy, passion, and professionalism, and a brand is built with *you* at its center — you are your brand. If your niche is working with bodybuilders, exercising like a bodybuilder and having the physical appearance of a bodybuilder will increase your brand. If you're a swimmer, swim. If you're a runner, run. If you're into yoga, do yoga. Appearing as part of a niche starts with living the part and looking the part.

Additionally, it's important to keep yourself healthy, keep yourself in shape. In-person personal training means you have to be there in person, healthy. Clients don't want to train with a sick personal trainer. Clients don't want to work with somebody who looks disheveled or appears dirty. Clients want somebody presentable: a professional and a mentor that will guide them in your particular area of expertise. Remember, you are an expert and a professional that brings value to your clients' lives — live your brand and be your brand.

As with personal training science and program design, there are many good books to help you understand business, sales and marketing. For additional reading, I recommend the following books:

Business Books

- *Good to Great* by James C. Collins
- *The Art of War* of Sun Tzu
- *The Lean Startup* by Eric Ries
- *The Power of Habit* by Charles Duhigg
- *Smarter Faster Better* by Charles Duhigg

Sales and Marketing Books

- *Contagious: Why Things Catch On* by Jonah Berger
- *They Ask You Answer* by Marcus Sheridan
- *Guerilla Marketing* by Jay Conrad Levinson
- *The Content Code* by Mark W. Schaefer
- *Hug Your Haters* by Jay Baer

- *Youtility* by Jay Baer
- *To Sell Is Human* by Daniel H. Pink
- *Pitch Anything* by Oren Klaff
- *How to Win Friends and Influence People* by Dale Carnegie

There are thousands more business, sales and marketing books out there with great information. Find your niche, find your passion and dive into the topics.

Note: I don't have any partnerships with the aforementioned books. Please refer to the Recommended Reading section for more details on the listed titles.

Personal trainers are overwhelmed by the amount of information there is in the industry. There are countless books, tools, materials and equipment produced. My goal in this chapter is to give you the foundational tools necessary to do your job and become successful in a short period of time. Next, we'll take these tools and apply them to your life, integrating them into your business so you can bring greater value to your clients and in doing so make more money.

Chapter Six

Integrating Your Tools

"Goals and objectives are based on theories and foundations."
-Abdolkarim Soroush-

"The question you need to ask yourself, is 'How much am I willing to work to achieve my goals?'"

As soon as Luke spoke those words, he knew he had been speaking to himself. He had been running a Heart Health group exercise session. Ted had partnered with a nutritionist and together they were offering a special lifestyle changing course for clients that were at risk of developing heart problems. The class had gone well, but there were a few members that weren't applying themselves and were feeling despondent. Luke had been giving them a motivational talk, but ended up motivating himself.

It had been a long couple of weeks, and he was feeling exhausted. However, Ted had kept on encouraging him. After giving him the templates and the forms to read and memorize, Ted took him to the next level. He said, "Having the theory and materials to be a good personal trainer is just the foundation towards achieving your goals. Anybody can have the materials, but it's about incorporating the materials into your everyday life and business that sets you up for success." Ted knew what it took to be successful, he had applied it in his own life and now he was mentoring Luke and guiding him along the path towards achieving his goals.

Luke had diligently looked inside himself, discovered his limitations and stepped through his fears. He had realized that his passion was personal training, and he had a deep motivation to help people and bring value to their lives. Ted had now begun to focus in on Luke's future plans.

"You have to put a plan in place, Luke. You can read about the tools, but never use them. You can read about how to set up a business, but never set one up. If you don't put the plan down in writing, you won't have the actual steps you need to take to succeed. *Be intentional about every decision you make, don't leave your success to chance.*" Ted spoke earnestly, he wanted Luke to realize the importance of planning; of having focus and direction. He continued, "Here is my original business plan, and here is my current business plan. I update this plan every six months. When I started personal training, I spent a lot of time feeling aimless. I was training people every day, but I didn't feel as if I was moving towards success or a goal. Once I wrote down my business plan, it focused me and gave me a vision. I want you to find your focus and have a vision."

The original business plan was handwritten and very basic. But Luke could see the value in the activity. Ted had defined his vision, his mission and his objectives. It gave him a written record of where he wanted to be and how he was going to get there — like stepping stones on a pathway.

"I never thought that a business plan could be so practical. I always had the impression that it was an unnecessary piece of admin that investors or bank managers require. But here you have 'action steps.' Did you actually take these steps, Ted?"

"Well, that's the funny thing about steps. When you are following a pathway of stepping stones, you have to physically step on each stone to reach your destination. It's the same with setting up a business, you have to complete each activity and step to move you towards your vision."

"It just seems like a lot of work…"

"It is a lot of work, but it's in the doing that you set up your success. The question you have to ask yourself is, 'How hard am I willing to work?'"

***

> "Focused, real hard work is the key to success. Keep your eyes on the goal, and just keep taking the next step towards completing it. If you aren't sure which way to do something, do it both ways and see which works better."
> -John Carmack-

In the previous section, you were given many tools. However, they're not useful until you integrate and implement them into your career and life. Without integration and implementation, this material is as flat as the other fitness industry books and certifications. They leave you stranded and without personal meaning.

In this section, you'll be taking the tools you've just learned and applying them to your individual situation. The reason why this is beneficial is because by doing so you will be reducing the gap for failure. If I just told you the science, gave you exercises or provided basic information around program design, you could be an average personal trainer with moderate success — maybe. However, by giving you activities to perform, I'm teaching you to *apply* the tools in a way that works for you and that gives the material personal meaning.

Do I still have your attention?

The other day, I was chatting with my driver about Unstoppable and he shared the following story, "I'm a certified personal trainer too! After I got my certification, I went to my local gym to apply for a position, but as I walked around and watched the other trainers, they were talking with their clients too much. I don't want to do that. I just want to get in, personal train, show my clients the exercises and get out."

Pay close attention – this is *not* personal training. Personal training is more than delivering exercises. If you just want to give your clients exercises, buy them an exercise book or direct them to one of the hundreds of exercise libraries available. (For example, www.ExRx.net)

So why do personal trainers still have jobs? We still have jobs because personal training is *more* than a mechanism for exercise delivery. Personal training is more than an exercise program and more than the latest health fad. Personal training is about coming alongside a client and making a difference in their lives. The value that you bring to improving their physical health and wellbeing will have a positive influence on every aspect of their lives.

How much are you willing to work?

You need to ask yourself, "How much am I willing to work to achieve my goals?" If you're not at the level you want to be, if your single session price is not what it could be, if your income doesn't equal your value, if you haven't taken the leap to become a gym owner or independent personal trainer, then you're not working smart enough.

Walk over to a mirror and take a long look at yourself. Lose the excuses because they aren't serving your purpose anymore. It's time to strap in because you're about to refocus your energy towards success.

In the previous chapter, all you did was *read* about tools that will make you successful. I am not letting you off that easy again. This section is riddled with activities that will make you stop and take immediate action towards creating success in your personal training career. In the appendix is an Activity Checklist where you can keep track of the completed activities.

COMPLETE EVERY ACTIVITY

Skipping exercises might have been your old actions, but this is a new you. The successful you. Grab a pad of paper, get some pens, and stretch out your hands because this is going to be a lot of essential work.

BUILDING ON YOUR FOUNDATION

In this section, I'll discuss how to set up different parts of your business using the tools we learned before. I'll first discuss how to set up everything you'll need to become a personal trainer. Next, I'll describe how to get started with marketing and sales. Lastly, I'll discuss how to set up a successful business.

If you're a new personal trainer, each section will benefit you. If you're an experienced personal trainer, there may be some parts that are more beneficial than others. There may be some areas that you didn't fully take advantage of when originally establishing your career, which is hurting your overall success.

Almost like a symptom of an injury or disease, people usually focus on the referred pain. The same is true when setting up your business — people often don't associate the referred pain (i.e. sales) with the deep problem (i.e. successful business setup). Read carefully and fix the actual issues.

Launching Your Personal Training Career

To set up your personal training career, it's important to understand the certifications and determine where you want to work. Without an initial plan in place, success is hard to find. Be intentional about every decision you make, whether it's about the certification you obtain, choosing to work for a gym, or starting your own business. Do not leave your success to chance, or you may be waiting a while.

Getting certified

A certification is not mandatory to be a personal trainer. Let me repeat myself, a certification is NOT a requirement to be a personal trainer. Only 89% of personal trainers hold a personal training certification in the US. Now, what does this say about personal trainers? It says you can develop personal training skills outside of the certification and still be a part of the community.

Certifications are incomplete because they do not build all the necessary skills to become successful. I've known personal trainers who didn't start with a certification, or haven't renewed their certifications because it's unnecessary and there's a knowledge gap in the certification programs. I am not strictly advocating to forego a certification because getting one will make it easier to get a gym interview and will establish respect with clients. However, what I am saying is that you *can* be successful without a certification or without continuously renewing your certification. You can be intelligent, you can understand how to train a client, you can be a great salesperson and you can be successful without a certification. That being said, I'll provide a quick overview of popular certification so you have a basic understanding of your options.

The gold standard certification in our industry is the NSCA's certification, and it's the one I obtained. NASM (National Academy of Sports Medicine) and ACSM (American College of Sports Medicine) are also very good certifications, while ACE (American Council on Exercise) is popular amongst new personal trainers (it was my first certification too!). There are other certification bodies out there, such as the ISSA (International Sports Sciences Association), however, they're not as popular, so we'll focus on these four for now.

Any of the certifications previously mentioned will cost hundreds of dollars, and hundreds more to renew when you take into account the CEU's (Continuing Education Units). The fitness industry requires personal trainers to pay for every step we take and the certification system was designed to make sure we all pay on a regular basis.

I am not against education; in fact, education is one of my highest priorities. I have multiple certifications, I've read dozens of fitness books and attended fitness events because I love learning so much. But you do not have to continuously pay certification renewal fees to be a successful personal trainer. You can be successful without CEU's or renewing your certification. Do what's right for you.

All ranting aside, if I were to rank the certifications based on my experience, the success of other personal trainers, industry feedback, and value, I would select the following order:

1. NSCA - #1 but also the hardest certification test. You need to have a degree in a science-related field to take the test.
2. NASM – large breadth of knowledge in science, program creation, business and more. I rank this just above ASCM because of the specialty CEU courses.
3. ACSM – large breadth of knowledge in science, program creation, business and more.
4. ACE – basic and useful for new personal trainers. It's also the most affordable certification of the four.

To keep a certification active, you need to receive CEU's. There are many ways to earn CEU's, including the following: attending industry events, attending seminars at local gyms, attending online courses, writing a book, speaking at an event, and so on.

Personal trainers who continue their education and find a passion for their career perform much better than those who don't. This is not in contradiction to my earlier statements. Learning for growth and creating knowledge on your own time is different to forced continuing education.

Find your passion, reach out to successful trainers who share your passion, follow the guidelines in this book and create success for yourself.

Activity: *Choose a certification to acquire.*

Where to work

There are many work opportunities where you can be successful as a personal trainer. There is no *one* successful path, which is a good thing. As I've repeated many times before, the best place to start is to know what you want and what you need.

What does this mean? If you're the type of person who does best when they're around other like-minded individuals, perhaps working for an employer (i.e. a gym) is best for you. Other personal trainers can help you gain experience, may be able to mentor you, and transfer knowledge quickly. Additionally, an employer will do basic marketing (though most gyms are mediocre at marketing). However, you'll also have less autonomy (control) and your employer will take a cut from your wages.

"Employer" is a very broad term, so I'll give it some definition now. An employer can be any number of institutions who are paying you to be a personal trainer — big box gyms, private studios, specialty gyms (i.e. boxing, TRX), universities, sports teams, hospitals and physical therapy clinics. There are many types of facilities to be an employee and there are tradeoffs for each institution type.

Another aspect of working at a gym, is that many gyms will give part-time personal trainers (<30 hours/week) a smaller percentage of the session revenue than full-time employee's (≥30 hours/week).

For example, a part-time personal trainer who is valued at $100/session may only make $30/session, whereas a full-time personal trainer at the same rate may make $50/session. There are many reasons why a gym wants the personal trainer to work full-time and earn the higher wage, but do be aware that employers take a large cut from your paycheck (most of the time). There may also be a ramp-up period, while working for an employer, before you achieve the higher pay scale. Understand the employer you want to work for and how much money you're willing to give up.

There's a tradeoff to being an employee versus an independent personal trainer. I want you to be knowledgeable in your decision-making process so you can be successful. Independent trainers receive 100% of the session price (special cases below).

The difficulties of being independent include more work in business setup, marketing, sales, and creating a prospect list. A gym usually takes care of the business management (including insurance), marketing, and sales operations, however, the independent personal trainer must own *all* aspects of the business. There's opportunity for success in each career path, it just depends on your values, strengths, and what you want and need.

Independent personal trainers have a few special cases where they do not earn 100% of the money from a session. There are some studios that provide a physical space and equipment so personal trainers can rent (reducing costs) and train their clients. Additionally, online personal training companies will ask for a percentage of each online session or charge a monthly service fee to use their software and client lists. Both are valid avenues to success.

Now it's a perfect time to discuss gym ownership. You've read the benefits and disadvantages for employees and independent personal trainers. As a prospective gym owner, use your new knowledge behind the advantages/disadvantages of different personal trainer employee types to market to personal trainers. There are also many avenues of gym ownership, such as franchising, launching a large-scale gym, private studio, specialty gym (i.e. kickboxing, yoga), or renting space to personal trainers. As I've repeated many times before, the best place to start is to know what you want and what you need. I'll provide additional information for prospective gym owners in the upcoming sections.

Activity: Select where you want to work.

Create basic 6-month exercise programs used during prospect sale pitches

In the next section of this book, I'll discuss how to create your own exercise programs. But first, I'll teach you a quick program creation method that will help set you up for the next section and will assist with your sales pitch (detailed in a later section).

You already have the exercise templates that I outlined in a previous section where I list workouts for seven days. Simply copy this program and create a 6-month calendar with the same exercises. At the end of the 6-months, you'll want to reassess your clients to compare against where they started and discuss new goals (if applicable).

Activity: *Create a 6-month calendar for all the provided exercise templates and any additional exercise templates you created yourself.*

Group training

Group training is a very effective way for personal trainers to earn more money with small (2 to 5 clients) and large groups (6 to 30 clients). Large group fitness training is outside the scope of this book, however, personal trainers can take the knowledge from this book to begin a basic group training career, or use it to supplement their personal training careers.

As with personal training, there are specific niches a group fitness trainer can select, as well as many certifications. Again, this is outside the scope of this book, so I'll focus on personal trainers who want to take their knowledge and apply it to larger groups.

In a previous section, I talked about setting up a business, sales, and marketing. To establish group training, you can still use all the information outlined before, you'll just need to update your marketing and sales to reflect the change in services offered and the associated prices.

Additionally, your niche will influence the type of exercise program you select such as following a weight loss exercise template. You may not need to use meal templates, however, it could be a successful benefit that isn't provided by many other large group trainers.

Most group trainers do not perform an initial consultation or physical assessment, but if you work at a gym, then it's expected that the assessments have been previously completed. However, it's still important for your group training clients to fill out the PAR-Q (and Medical Release Form if necessary), Referral Form, and Client Session Sign-in Sheet (with every session).

Group training can provide much more money than one hour of personal training. Group trainers frequently price their services at a quarter to a third of the price of a one-on-one training session for each group client and host 6 to 30 clients in a group. When added together, this can translate to up to ten times more money for a group session compared to a one-on-one training session. This is where you can make a lot of money, increase the visibility of your brand, and receive a high amount of referrals.

However, it's also important to understand one of the most difficult parts of group training – maintaining a personal connection. Depending on a group's size, it's difficult to provide a personalized connection with each member because during a group training session you have many responsibilities: communicating the exercise, observing form, gauging difficulty level, providing exercise progressions/regressions, setting up the next exercise, and connecting with individuals.

Launch Your Business

Personal trainers typically understand basic sciences and common training tools. It's been my experience that you don't need to have deep scientific knowledge to have success. However, you do need to understand how to set up a business to be successful and, unfortunately, this is where our industry and certification programs do a poor job of imparting knowledge.

Where do you start? What do you do? You may have jumped into personal training because you love fitness, but the truth is passion alone will only take you so far. Without an understanding of business fundamentals, you're going to fail. Sit down, pay attention, and get ready to build your business.

Selecting Your Niche

Throughout this book, you've identified your passions, values, and goals, and now it's time to determine your niche (target) fitness market. What type of fitness do you enjoy? Who do you like to help (for example, the elderly)? Answering these questions will help create your niche and find the types of clients you'll target with your business. Popular niches include working with weight loss goals, focusing on the elderly, working with athletes or building strength.

Creating a focused niche is important in order to achieve success faster. Your business needs to be focused so that your community understands your services and is able to differentiate you from your competitors. Without a focused niche, every other personal trainer is your competitor. With a focused niche, you have fewer competitors, you gain expertise within that niche, and it's easier to receive referrals from other personal trainers who cannot service specific clients.

When defining your niche, it's also important to consider industry trends. What's popular today may not be in the future and understanding trends can determine how you sell your services. Most personal trainers do not adapt to changing industry trends, which is one of the reasons why most trainers are not successful. Remember that creating a business means selling a product that people want; if you don't consider the changing attitudes of the industry, your business will not remain successful for long. I want you to be successful in the present and the future, so please pay attention to fluctuating industry patterns.

So what are some industry trends today? Below is a list of current fitness industry trends, which will help create your niche:

- Increase in specialty gyms such as MMA, TRX, boxing, kickboxing, dance, yoga, pilates, stationary bikes, etc.
- HIIT workouts
- Prevalence of strength, circuit, and bodyweight training
- Group training (6 to 30 clients)
- Group personal training (2 to 5 clients)
- Outdoor activities such as hiking, rock climbing, parkour

- Flexibility and mobility training
- Exercise as a form of preventative health such as lowering the risk of heart disease, stroke, cancer, dementia, and other chronic diseases
- Fitness programs for older adults. As adults age (the Baby Boomer generation), more businesses are focusing their services on this huge market
- Functional training, which focuses on training for daily activities, such as moving furniture, sitting at a desk, carrying a toddler, and walking with a briefcase
- Gym memberships are increasing
- In America, nearly 70% of people over 20 are overweight including those who are obese. This statistic allows for many personal trainers to concentrate on weight loss programs
- Technology is increasingly making its way into fitness – wearable technology, online fitness videos and streaming, online personal training
- Number and types of personal training certifications – this may have an effect on a prospective client's perception of personal trainers who do not have a certification
- Worksite health promotion where companies create programs to advocate positive health choices, with some companies building on-site fitness facilities and providing professional-led workshops for their employees
- Wellness coaching, which is full-service coaching focused on increasing somebody's strengths and finding satisfaction in life

Activity: *Select your niche.*

Three types of personal trainers

There are three main types of in-person personal trainers –

employee, independent personal trainer, and business owner. What personal trainer type will you be? This all depends on your goals and the type of services you want to provide your community, which depends on your niche (see the previous section). Below is a list of benefits and disadvantages for each personal trainer type:

Employee (gym, private studio, community center, etc.)

- The benefits of being an employee are many and include the following free materials: marketing (i.e. website, physical picture posted), branding (associate you with gym culture), prospect list (gym members), branded t-shirt, potential successful personal training mentors and resources (i.e. fitness equipment)
- The disadvantages are the following: reduced paycheck, limited prospects, and limited control

Independent personal trainer

- The benefits of being an independent trainer include: control (schedule, price), leadership, location flexibility and creating your own brand
- The disadvantages are the following – traveling to locations, you have to juggle all aspects of a business (i.e. liability), you have to manage your marketing (attracting prospects, social media), you're always hustling, and you have to purchase your own materials (i.e. fitness equipment)

Business owner

- The benefits of being a business owner include: control (schedule, price, brand, employees), leadership, you can create your own brand, management (might enjoy), and you can make money through employees even when you're not working.

- The disadvantages are the following: management (you may not get to personal train anymore), you have to juggle all aspects of a business (i.e. liability), you have to manage the marketing (attracting prospects, social media), and you're always hustling.

Some of you will be able to select more than one personal trainer type. For example, some gyms let you train inside and outside their gym. Other gyms have a strict policy against letting you train outside their gym. You have to choose between their gym and working independently. The choice is yours.

Activity: Select your preferred trainer type.

Location

One of the highest determiners of business success is location. One of the benefits of being an independent personal trainer is your location isn't fixed – you can travel to clients; and, personal training employees succumb to the success of a gym's location. Where will you set up?

PROSPECTIVE GYM OWNERS, pay attention – location matters to your market. The best place to start is with research on demographic and economic data (i.e. American FactFinder, state data centers, economic census), which will help determine where people live, work, and spend money. Additionally, it's imperative you do competitive research to find out what your competition is doing, such as how or where they're succeeding and failing, so that you avoid a flooded market and can find your own route to success. You have much more work to do than the other personal trainer types.

Activity: Select your business location.

Setting Your Price

There are multiple ways to set the price for your personal training services and we cover the following price techniques:

Market Rate, Bundle, Fixed, Fluid, and two Bonus Advanced techniques.

Let's dive into the various ways that personal trainers sell their services.

Market Rate

Each geographical location will have a different average personal training session price range, also known as the market rate. The best references to set your prices are to research. Ask personal trainers, go to gyms, research on Yelp, factor in the economics of your niche and discover your local price range.

In addition to research, setting your price requires strategic thinking. Some of you may find it beneficial to set your price similar to the other trainers in your area. As a new trainer, you may choose to set the price slightly lower to get a small competitive edge, until you grow your daily client session count.

Likewise, if the average local personal training session is $50/hour, but your clients have a track record of achieving their goals faster or more consistently, your value is higher than the average personal trainer, which means your single session price should be higher than average.

Bundle

There are multiple ways to sell your services. A popular technique is to set a high single session cost and reduce the session price with large session bundles. For example, if I set my price at $50 for a single session, I may set a five session training bundle at $200. The client will be more inclined to purchase the bundle because the single session price is lower. Purchasing the five session bundle at $200 ($40/session) is more affordable than purchasing five single sessions for $250 (5 sessions x $50 = $250). Creating session bundles commits the client, gives more time to show your value, increases the likelihood for repeat business, and creates a long-term revenue stream.

Additionally, bundles come in various sizes and I've seen them go as high as 30 sessions. The bundle sizes that have worked best for me have been 5, 10 and 20 sessions. Moreover, bundles do *not* have to be discounted but 95% of personal training bundles are discounted, so choose wisely.

Clients will more often purchase a bundle than single sessions. Understanding this idea gives you an additional pricing option – inflating your per session prices. You now know clients opt for bundles over single sessions. You also know it's industry standard to decrease the price of a session when purchased in a bundle. Understanding both of these ideas allows you to work the system – you can increase your single session price to provide additional income.

For example, your current single session price is $50 and a five session bundle is $40 per session. Inflating your price may increase your single session from $50 to $60 (20% increases) and five session bundle from $40 to $50 (25% increase) per session.

Lastly, there are many benefits to push bundles over a single session, including:

- Clients are more committed
- Clients can afford the bundle price now but may not in the future (you can always switch to single sessions if necessary)
- You won't have to collect money as often

Fixed vs. Fluid

Fixed pricing is popular at institutions (i.e. gyms) and with inexperienced personal trainers because it's simpler for marketing and sales to have flat rates. A fixed price (aka flat rate) is setting the same price for all clients, goals, and outcomes.

For example, you set a fixed rate of $50/session for two clients – a 40-year-old male who has never worked out and wants to lose 50 pounds in a year, and a 20-year-old female athlete who wants to increase her upper body strength.

Fluid pricing is popular amongst more experienced personal trainers because it permits pricing flexibility, allowing for increased prices for more complex clients.

For example, your rate for a 20-year-old female athlete who wants to increase her upper body strength is $50/session but is $60 for the 40-year-old male who has never worked out and wants to lose 50 pounds in a year.

Choose Fixed or Fluid pricing based on your comfort level. If you choose to go with Fluid pricing and you're wondering how to market your services, you can list prices as a range, such as "between $50 and $60" or list the lowest amount, such as "As low as $50 a session."

BONUS: Advanced Price Techniques

Outcome-based

I've used this technique in the past with great success because clients are purchasing an outcome. Outcome-based pricing is a clever marketing technique that doesn't provide much additional direct value to your client, but it identifies more with a client's goals and provides intrinsic value. Either way, you sell more packages (aka bundles) and the client feels a greater commitment to their goals. Outcome-based pricing means developing bundles around specific goals, or outcomes.

For example, instead of naming your bundles Beginner, Intermediate, and Advanced, you can use outcome-based naming to create Healthy Back, Build Muscle, and Fat Loss for Swimsuit Season.

Do you see how the outcome-based bundles quickly communicate and connect you to the services provided? I highly suggest the outcome-based pricing technique.

Recurrent Value

One of the smartest pricing conventions is to receive recurrent income from client training. Recurrent (aka repeated) pricing moves away from single sessions and bundle systems to a monthly payment system.

Let's think about this — if your sales strategy includes a single session or bundle-based system, write down the number of sessions a client trains per month and any other direct services. You're most likely offering clients a one-on-one training session, the fitness program where you're pulling each individual session, possibly a nutrition plan and a nutrition journal. These are the activities and materials a client interacts with directly.

In addition, there are indirect activities and materials provided, such as the time it takes to write the program, the time it takes to adjust a program to daily needs, progressing or regressing short and long-term goals, and a program for traveling or when on holiday.

In the recurrent pricing model, you take all the indirect activities, place a price tag on them, and charge your clients on a continuous basis. Let's run through an example of both models below.

Familiar price per session example:

You price a single session at $50 and work with a client 2x/week. In a month, they are seeing you for 8 sessions (4 weeks x 2 sessions/week), and if purchased on an individual session basis, you would make $400/month from this client. Understand the client can cancel a session in this model, so your revenue can fluctuate depending on your client's whims.

Recurrent pricing example:

You price a single session at $50 and work with a client 2x/week. In a month, they are seeing you for eight sessions (4 weeks x 2 sessions/week), which is $400/month. Now, you add in your indirect activities at $50/month. This brings you up to $450/month for one client.

Instead of receiving $50/session which is subject to client

availability, you're receiving a steady stream of $450/month, which isn't subject to change. Additionally, you can easily show your client the $450/month value you bring to them, and then discount the monthly price to $375/month, not subject to change based on the client's availability. You provide much more value than your clients see, whether it's advice, motivation, or travel programs. You should be compensated for your work.

Understand what you want, your value, what you're willing to do in order to succeed, your strengths and your weaknesses. Understand the level you're at today and the level you want to be in your future. Know your value and set your price based on the services you can offer your clients.

Activity: *Select your pricing model.*

Set Up Your Business Plan

Uh-oh, a business plan? You may be looking at this section with anxiety thinking of all the work you need to put in. You're right, it can be difficult to write a business plan. But guess what? If you've taken the time to read the previous sections and do the exercises, you've already completed some of the work! Additionally, business plans can serve many purposes, which means they vary in detail. If you're an employee, you don't need a business plan, though it's wise to understand business creation basics for your future.

I've written many business plans, short and long, for companies I've started and been employed at. These documents are necessary and are an organized projection of what you want your business to be.

If you're an independent trainer, you can most likely get away with a condensed business plan that outlines the basics of your business. A shortened business plan might cover the following information:

- Vision – What are you building? What will your business look like in the future (i.e. 1-year, 3-years)?

- Mission – Why are you starting this business? What is the purpose?
- Objectives – Create S.M.A.R.T. goals for your business. How will you measure success in achieving your goals?
- Strategies – What will you sell? How will you sell? What makes you different to the others?
- Startup Capital – How much money will you need to launch your business?
- Anticipated Expenses – What are the estimated monthly costs of running your business in months 1, 3, 6, and 12?
- Desired Income – What do you anticipate your monthly income will be in months 1, 3, 6, and 12?
- Action Plan – What are the task items you need to complete today? To reach future milestones?

If you're a prospective gym owner or you're starting any other type of fitness company (i.e. product sales), then you want a detailed business plan. Business plans are essential because they help qualify your business idea, are necessary for financing (bank loan, investors), and provide detailed information on background and budget. Many unsuccessful personal trainers fail to write a business plan – do you think there's a correlation?

The traditional, longer business plan has the following sections:

- Executive Summary – An overview of the business plan which highlights the most important information. This section is typically written last.
- Company Description – Location, company size, vision and mission, services and purpose.
- Services – What you're selling and the value you bring to your clients.
- Market Analysis – Detailed overview of the industry, and an outline of your target market and competition.

- Marketing Strategy - Outlines how your business fits into the market and how you'll price, promote, and sell your services.
- Management Summary – Structure of business, who's involved, and how it's managed.
- Financial Analysis (most difficult part) – Details the financing of your business today, what's required for growth, and your operating expenditures.

The business plans get detailed quickly, but remember we've outlined many of the questions and answers in the previous sections. Think that was an accident?

Activity: *Create your business plan*

Fund your business

As we saw in the Financial Analysis section in the business plan, this may be the hardest part of starting your business. If you're an independent personal trainer, funding your business might not require much effort. However, pay attention to the details below and save yourself time and money. For all of those entrepreneurs launching a gym and need real financing, read on.

How will you start your business? If you don't have money to launch a business yourself, you'll need to raise or borrow funds to open up your dream gym. After you determine how much money you'll need, use the most appropriate information below:

- Self-funding – Ask family or friends for money, use your savings, or tap into your 401k (keep complete control of the business).
- Investment – Money is exchanged for ownership and an active role in the company. Visit your local US Small Business Administration (SBA) office for advice – I've used them and received great advice.
- Crowdfunding – Money is obtained without giving up ownership. However, crowdfunders expect to get a gift,

product, service, or credit in return. This is a low-risk version of funding.

- Small-business loan – Keep full control of your business with a loan, through banks or credit unions.

Activity: *List the type of funding you will prioritize.*

Set up Successful Business Operations

Selecting a **business structure** is extremely important because it determines the way you can operate and outlines different business burdens, such as tax payments and liability. The different business structure types include: sole proprietorship, general partnership, limited liability company (LLC), corporation, or a combination of these. Selecting a business structure is outside the scope of this book, however, the SBA has great resources on selecting what's right for you.

Selecting a **business name** may sound easy, but it can get complex quickly. You need to select a business name that works for you, but also realize it affects other parts of your business, such as: website domain name (doesn't have to match business name), trademark (review USPTO website), and entity name (protects at the state level).

Set up an **employer identification number (EIN)**, which is a federal tax number specific to your business and is required if you will have employees or plan to form a partnership, LLC, or corporation. You can use the IRS website to receive your EIN.

Obtain a **business license** using your EIN from the previous step, which is a mandatory license to run your business. A business license is strongly recommended for all business owners including independent personal trainers.

If you are opening a physical location, you may need to fill out a **business personal property tax** form. This form is used for taxes when purchasing tangible personal property.

There may be additional **licenses and permits** depending on your state, so I highly recommend reaching out to the SBA to help you out.

I strongly recommend opening a **business bank account** and keeping expenditures separate from your personal funds. If not, you may have trouble with the IRS in the future. Reach out to your bank or local credit union to set up an account.

Set up an **accounting system** (e.g. Excel, QuickBooks) to help manage your finances. It will make your life much easier come tax season.

Activity: *Complete each task in the successful business operations section and develop all branded tools from the previous section.*

Sound Business Practices

The most important business practice to adopt is the following – create happiness, daily. Create happiness for yourself and you'll thrive. Create happiness in your business and it will flourish. Create happiness for your clients, and they will return again and again.

Additionally, treat everyone (client, prospect, and stranger) as a part of your brand, part of your family. Developing a strong brand creates a strong community and should be a focus at all times, whether it's during marketing, sales, client onboarding, client sessions, industry events, or meeting new people outside of work.

A strong community creates strong bonds with people and they'll feel like family. For example, with a strong brand, clients are walking billboards boasting about your skills, and even become brand ambassadors – giving you referrals and positive reviews verbally and digitally.

Moreover, to develop a strong brand it's important to establish baseline rules that will make you and your clients successful. It's important to set rules for your clients. Creating rules helps establish a baseline of respect and professionalism that your clients will appreciate. What are your rules? Some rules that I suggest are:

- 24-hour cancellation policy – Without this in place, clients may take advantage of canceling sessions on a whim which hurts your bottom line, and the value you can provide
- Clients must wear athletic clothes
- Clients must bring water
- Clients must notify you of updated physical concerns, nutritional information and changing schedules
- Clients must carry, and inform you, of required health accouterments such as Epileptic pens, snacks for low blood sugar, etc.

It's also important to set rules for yourself. Creating rules commits you to professionalism and daily success, which will be appreciated by your clients, coworkers, and employees (for the gym owners out there). What do you need on a daily basis to be successful? Some rules I suggest are:

- I will personal train five or more clients a day unless I'm on vacation or sick
- I will not show up to a session unprepared
- I will not be late to personal training sessions

Activity: *Write rules for yourself and your clients.*

Launch Your Sales and Marketing

If you've developed the sales and marketing tools from the previous section, you're in a good position. To set up your sales and marketing efforts, the easy part is you only have to focus on developing your prospect list. The difficult part is that you have to focus on developing your prospect list.

I previously discussed the benefits of working for an employer in that you're typically given a prospect list to kick-off your career. For all you other personal trainers, it's time to get to work. Developing your prospect list takes discipline, consistency, and enthusiasm.

Business cards will develop your prospect list slowly because you typically hand out your card on an individual in-person basis. Flyers are more widespread but get a mixed reception – many people toss flyers immediately without ever reading the material.

The most effective ways to develop your prospect list are through digital marketing (networking) and referrals.

Digital marketing comes in the form of your website, professional sites, review sites, and social media. Your website is one of your best tools because you control the message for your prospects. You get the opportunity to talk about your services, your brand, what sets you apart, and to deliver immediate value.

Creating a **website** is simpler than ever before, and it can take as little as a few hours. You can use GoDaddy to register your website and WordPress to select a simple website framework. Afterwards, inputting pictures and writing your business content is the fun part. Remember to include a Contact Me page so there's a way for your prospects to get in touch with you, enabling the development of your prospect list.

Create a profile on **professional sites** so that you develop your brand's presence. Creating a profile on many different professional sites can increase your digital visibility. I highly recommend starting with LinkedIn because it can help you network with many people. To a lesser extent, I suggest joining fitness communities and become an active participant, helping people with your professional opinion and advice. I suggest joining Endomondo, Strava, Traineo, Runkeeper, DailyBurn or FitLink.

Developing a presence on **review sites** is an easy way to accumulate testimonials and success stories for your business.

Additionally, review sites are another way for prospects to come into contact with your business, and a positive review increases your sales (aka conversion rate). I highly recommend creating a profile on Yelp and Zomato, and begin writing reviews as a fitness professional. Additionally, ask friends, family, and coworkers to write positive reviews about your business on Yelp, Foursquare, and TripAdvisor.

There are many benefits to **social media** and none truer than you get to spread your brand in creative ways. I recommend using Facebook, Instagram, YouTube, Twitter, Pinterest, Periscope, and Snapchat. Use what works best for you, spread your brand awareness, and increase your prospect list.

Referrals are a great place to start your prospect list. You want to begin by asking family, friends, and coworkers to provide referrals for your business. You can start by asking directly or you can offer the referrers free sessions so they feel there's a value trade — a win/win situation. Referrals are the best source of prospect generation because they provide an extra layer of trust for the prospect. This makes the referred person a more prized prospect because they are more willing to purchase your services (aka they're known as a qualified prospect or lead).

Activity: *Set up your digital marketing, reach out for referrals, and develop all tools from the previous section.*

BONUS: In-Person Daily Brand Checklist

In addition to the marketing and sales ideas outlined earlier, you want to have a daily in-person brand checklist (a plan to help increase the visibility of your business) in place so that you're creating a professional and positive environment. Here are a few ideas for your checklist:

- Confirm appointments with clients prior to their first few sessions — in addition to creating a professional environment, this added benefit allows clients to easily communicate updates on their health, such as injuries (physical), low blood sugar (nutrition), or a fight with a partner (emotional). In my experience, clients will still attend a training session without communicating their health needs, expecting you to be flexible enough to update their program on the fly. It's best to communicate early and be prepared

- Smile and say hello to everyone — every person is a prospect if they're not already a client. Even if you're at a gym, the employees of the gym are prospects. Other personal trainers are prospects. Everybody around you is a new opportunity to market and brand yourself. Every conversation not had is an opportunity missed
- Business cards — always have them in your pocket
- Business flyers — always have them in your bag, especially if you're an independent personal trainer

Activity: *Write your own daily brand checklist.*

PROSPECT SESSIONS – INITIAL CONSULTATION AND PHYSICAL ASSESSMENT

Personal training section

To integrate our personal training tools from the previous section, the best path forward is to walk through the prospect sessions including the initial consultation and physical assessment. The prospect sessions in many gyms are free sessions given to all members to help sell personal training (the highest grossing service at a gym).

There are two ways to split up the prospect sessions and they are: Two individual sessions (usually one hour each) or one aggregate session (the initial consultation plus physical assessment; the initial consultation paperwork will need to be completed by the prospect and sent to the personal trainer prior to this meeting). I've performed both session types and prefer meeting for two individual sessions. It gives more time to learn about the prospect, builds trust, and makes it easier to ask for the sale.

Initial consultation

An hour before the initial consultation, confirm the prospect is coming in to meet with you; this is usually accomplished with a quick mobile text message. Gather all your materials including the Client Intake Forms, Medical Release Form, Food Journal, and Client Session Sign-in Sheet.

Fifteen minutes before the initial consultation, make sure you're dressed appropriately using my previous recommendations, including: branded t-shirt, exercise clothing, and athletic shoes. Confirm you also have all necessary non-exercise equipment and a quiet space to meet with the prospect.

Two minutes before the initial consultation, arrive at the designated meeting location and gather your energy. Be yourself, stay focused, and come prepared to make a connection with the prospect. When the prospect arrives, introduce yourself and make your way to your predetermined quiet area. The initial consultation is your first opportunity to show value, build your brand, and sell yourself. I've provided much material, which you'll need to review with the prospect within this one hour. Begin by asking the prospect to use the client session sign-in sheet to check in for this session and provide an overview of the documents you'll fill out together over the next hour.

Additionally, I highly suggest learning the material well enough so you can have a conversation with the prospect and you're not just reading the forms' question lists. Having a conversation will feel much better for both of you, however, if you feel more comfortable reading the outlined forms, please do so. Remember that the PAR-Q section of the intake form needs to be treated seriously and may require you to get the prospect's physician to complete the Medical Release Form before proceeding with the physical assessment.

Moreover, the Food Journal is given to the prospect at the end of the initial consultation as homework and they are asked to fill out the form with 3 to 7 days of nutritional information (depending on your preference). You end the first session with an overview of the information addressed in the initial consultation, how it helps give a picture of their fitness goals, an overview of the upcoming physical assessment, Medical Release Form (if necessary), and you need to SET THE PHYSICAL ASSESSMENT APPOINTMENT, preferably within seven days of the initial consultation so your value stays top of their mind.

Physical assessment

An hour before the physical assessment, again confirm the prospect is coming in to meet with you. Gather all your materials including all the forms from the initial consultation, client session sign-in sheet, price sheet and physical assessment forms.

Fifteen minutes before the physical assessment, make sure you're dressed appropriately using the previous recommendations on professional attire. Confirm you also have the necessary exercise and non-exercise equipment, and a quiet space to meet with the prospect to review the material.

Two minutes before the fitness assessment, arrive at the designated meeting location and gather your energy. Be yourself, stay focused, and be prepared to connect with the prospect. When the prospect arrives, greet them and make your way to the predetermined quiet area. The goal of the physical assessment is to test the physical abilities of your prospect through movement. The physical assessment activities are outlined in the materials of the previous section and will take 30 – 60 minutes to complete.

The physical assessment is your second in-person opportunity to show value, build your brand, and sell yourself. You have much material to review with the prospect within this one hour. Begin by asking the prospect to use the Client Session Sign-in Sheet to check in, provide an overview of the physical assessment activities, review any open questions you may have from the initial consultation documents, and review their Food Journal. Try to complete the non-exercise activities in 15 minutes or less so you have enough time for the physical assessment and wrap-up conversation.

How do you build additional value during the fitness assessment?

Ask your client questions throughout each assessment activity, specifically to determine their comfort level with each exercise. It's also your job to take note of your prospect's movements, if they're having trouble with a movement (overall, specific muscles), and if they're struggling at any point (reduced breathing, red- faced, etc.).

For example, during the squat exercise assessment, if your prospect's upper torso leans too far forward, a few possible explanations are that their hip flexors are too tight or their back is too weak. What does identifying this information mean to the client? What does it mean to you? Your focus brings to light an added benefit to your services by discovering weaknesses, identifying issues they can't see themselves, and adding tasks to their fitness goals. The more (honest) value you can identify and bring in the initial consultation and physical assessment, the stronger the bond will be with the prospect and yourself. By creating more value and demonstrating that value, the prospect will be more inclined to buy services from you.

Additionally, you'll want to leave at least 15 minutes at the end of the physical assessment to review the prospect's results, review the basic 6-month proposed exercise program, review your price sheet and sell your services. Do not rush the closing remarks and sale, otherwise, the likelihood of a sale will be diminished. We'll review the art of selling in the next chapter

BONUS: Developing relationships to build your business

Personal training is not only about the long-term goals you set, the exercises you give to your prospects/clients, or the progressions and regressions to achieve their goals. Personal training is taking the tools at your disposal, the massive amounts of information you've gathered on the client, and integrating this knowledge into a plan that works for the individual. In its most basic level, personal training is about communication and empathy. Communicating the knowledge you have and empathizing with your client to adapt their program appropriately.

To become successful, you must change your mindset from providing sessions to strengthening the relationship you have with the client. If you do not care about effective communication, personal training is not your field.

If you do not care to ask about a client's personal life, you will not have a long- term relationship with them. Yes, each client is different and some will be more open to building a relationship and sharing than others. Be flexible enough to adapt to those clients that are talkers and to those that are more introverted. Be willing to learn about your clients and get to know them. Be prepared to *care* about your clients.

When you show you care, you're building a strong bond, you're building a brand, and you're building your reputation. You do this by understanding what your client needs.

So where do you get this information? You gather this information from each moment you spend with your client, starting with the initial consultation and their communication style throughout the fitness assessment and client sessions.

How does empathy make you successful professionally and financially? Empathizing with your clients shows that you're listening, understanding, and caring about your clients as individuals.

For example, if you have a client who's missing sessions because they're sick, you can still connect with the client and ask them how they are, if there's something you can provide, and send them health tips to assist them in recovering. (Communication outside of a fitness session is appreciated by most people, but not all; it's important to ask your clients if you can send them messages with health information.)

The more you know and understand your client, the more effective you can become in tailoring their program to meet their specific likes and dislikes, needs and goals. The more effective your program, the more motivated your client will be and the more successful that client will be in meeting those goals. This will have a positive effect on your success as a personal trainer, on your brand and on your professional reputation. By providing extra value to your clientele, you build stronger bonds that tie them to your brand and services longer, which means more money for you.

Want to sell?

Now that you've set up your business and you've gone over the initial prospect assessments, how do you get the person as a client? In the next part, I'll review how to get your first clients and kick-off your sales efforts.

Chapter Seven

Building on Your Success

"If you're interested in the living heart of what you do, focus on building things rather than talking about them."
- Ryan Freitas-

The telephone rang... Luke and Ted were in the office preparing the folders for that morning's clients. Luke was busy with Mary's folder, they were going to be reassessing her progress and adapting her program.

"Hi, Ted here, how can I help you?... Hi Jenna, oh no, I'm so sorry to hear that. Is she okay?" Ted looked concerned, "Well, at least she didn't break something. Please let me know if I can help with anything. Could you ask her if she would be okay with me sending her some health tips to recover? I know a few natural alternatives that can help with the bruising. Thanks Jenna, please tell her not to worry, we'll adapt her sessions for a bit. Would it be okay with you if I call the physical therapist to find out any details that I need to be aware of? Thanks, please keep me posted. I'll call tomorrow to see how she is. Take care. Bye," Ted put the phone down. He looked concerned.

"That was Mary's daughter. Mary had a fall over the weekend. She slipped on a wet tile and fell. The doctor said that if she'd had this fall a year ago, she would have been in hospital but because her balance and strength has improved so much, she managed to grab onto the counter to slow down the fall. She sprained her wrist and is bruised badly on the hip, but there are no fractures. She's just been to her physical therapist. She'll have to take it easy for a couple of days."

"I'm sorry to hear that. I'm glad she's okay. Is there anything we could do to help her?"

"Well, I think we can send her a fruit basket or some flowers to let her know we are thinking of her. She loves chocolates, but she's worked so hard on losing weight that I really want to encourage her to keep going with her diet and not see this as a setback. Then, we'll also have to adapt her program for a couple of weeks. She needs to rest for now, but at the same time, once she is up and about I'd like to get her back into her routine as soon as possible. I'm just going to give her therapist a call." Ted picked up the phone and left the office.

Luke was once more amazed at the care that Ted showed to his clients. Having worked with Ted for a while now, Luke's whole concept of personal training had been transformed. His focus had shifted from creating sessions to building relationships. He had come to realize that the personal training was more than just giving a client exercises and providing them with sessions. It was about journeying with them, genuinely caring for them and doing your best to make a difference in their lives. Ted went the extra mile with each of his clients. He didn't focus on making money, he focused on bringing value and making a difference.

And that's exactly what Ted had done in Luke's life. He had brought value and was making a difference in Luke's life, both current and future. Over the weeks, Ted had helped Luke start building his future business and brand. They had set up the business side of things, Ted had equipped him with sales and marketing skills and a toolkit of skills and knowledge. They had now started working on the actual personal training skills and integrating it all into successful, personalized programs for each client. Luke thought that he knew how to create an exercise program, how to adapt a meal plan and how to sell to clients. But Ted's step-by-step approach, based on his experience, had shown him otherwise.

As Luke paged through Mary's folder to find the plan for the session that they were supposed to have, he once more noticed the detailed templates and forms and how Ted had adapted each one according to Mary's specific needs. He noticed the extra little notes that Ted had made on Mary's preferences, including her love for chocolate, her battle with losing weight and a note to bring an extra water bottle because she kept forgetting hers. Ted had gone the extra mile and anticipated her needs for each session.

At the workout page for that day, Luke noticed that Ted had suggested exercises to Luke based on his knowledge of Mary. Ted, as always, had gone the extra mile and anticipated Luke's needs before he had even communicated them. It suddenly struck Luke, Ted had given him a key to successful personal training and to business — *go the extra mile*. He was determined to apply that in his sessions and in his business.

***

> "Embrace what you don't know, especially in the beginning, because what you don't know can become your greatest asset. It ensures that you will be doing things differently from everybody else."
> - Sara Blakely –

You've come so far. You've identified your goals, committed to a personal training career, created business tools, learned to apply the tools to your life, gathered prospects along the way and have performed the assessment sessions.

You've built a platform for success and it's time to claim your prize. Throughout this section, I'll teach you some of the last tools you'll need to be successful such as how to create an exercise program, different features of diet programs, and how to sell to your prospects!

This section is punctuated with important activities. If you complete the activities in this section (and throughout the book), you'll have gained up to 10 years in successful personal training knowledge.

Seize this opportunity and succeed immediately.

PERSONAL TRAINING

Now it's time to learn how to bring all the information you've gathered on your prospect and turn it into a successful *client* health program.

I'll start with describing how to build complete exercise and meal programs, and then I'll run through a client session. I'm giving you the tools to write your own programs so you can be successful today, and in the future. Learning to build your own programs is a necessary skill for all successful personal trainers. It allows you to easily produce personalized programs, adapt daily programs based on client energy levels, and understand the basic tools of your trade.

Stay focused and get ready to advance your skills on the path to success.

Building a Full Exercise Program

Exercises programs will differ in many facets including frequency, duration, and intensity. I'll describe the basics of all exercise programs and dive into specific training methods including a deep dive into a successful framework.

There is so much information available that it's hard to determine what, when, or why you'll do something. Throughout this section, I'll be as specific as possible without getting too deep. The goal of this section is to give you the basic tools to create your own exercise programs. If an idea or tool isn't familiar to you, please do further research to expand your understanding.

Let's get started.

As a general overview, here are the basics of an exercise program:

1. Soft tissue work (5 – 10 minutes)
2. Dynamic warm-up (5 – 15 minutes)
3. Main workout (20 – 40 minutes)
4. Stretching (10 – 15 minutes)

It's important to understand that for most clients who are just starting out with a workout program, they may only be able to complete soft tissue work, a dynamic warm-up and stretching, due to many reasons (eg. low energy levels). It's your job to focus on your client and understand their daily capabilities.

Soft tissue work

Soft tissue work is a great place to start any training program. Soft tissue work is expressed in many ways, but the most widely understood is massage. Massaging the soft tissue (muscle, fascia or connective tissue) helps the body in so many ways, including improving the quality of muscle, releasing tension and helping speed recovery. If you feel comfortable with massage, I highly recommend applying your skills to your clients.

Soft tissue work can be done before, during, or after a workout. If you don't know massage and don't have clients that can afford to regularly visit a massage therapist (99% of all clients), then it's best to begin a training session with foam rolling.

Foam rolling is an affordable version of massage and is also called self-myofascial release because the client is usually using a tool to release their own body's tension. The tools you can employ are foam rollers, tennis balls, lacrosse balls, and more. It's important to instruct the client to *not* foam roll over joints because it can apply too much pressure to sensitive areas or over bony parts because it can be uncomfortable and is unnecessary. Moreover, it will be harder for injured, overweight, and older clients to maneuver a foam roller. It's beneficial to take into account your client's specific needs.

For example, a client may not need to foam roll their quads every workout but may need more focus on their chest and hamstring. Each client is different, so pay attention and do what's right for your client.

Most clients will appreciate foam rolling the gluteal muscles, IT band, quads, calves, lats, and back. If you're unsure how to perform foam rolling, there are many instructional videos on YouTube.

Dynamic stretching

There are many types of stretching, but I've found dynamic stretching works best prior to a workout because it employs movement through a client's full range of movement, which increases internal body heat, loosens muscles, and prepares the body for most activities. As always, understand your clients and the best activities for their needs.

I've tried many dynamic warm-up exercises throughout my career and I find the best to be the following:

- Inchworm – full body movement
- Lunge walk (forward, backward, lateral)
- Lunge walk with a twist – helps to open up the legs and back
- Spiderman crawl
- Bear crawl
- Walking over and under – used by most collegiate and professional athletes to open the hips
- Walking knee lift
- Wall squats with a stability ball on the back – develops good squat technique while warming up the legs and core muscles
- Bridge (double- and single-leg) – helps activate the gluteal muscles which are typically deactivated (aka not fully or appropriately being used)
- Jumping jacks
- Skipping

Main workout

The main, or body, of a workout, is what many of you are anticipating. I highly recommend spending more time understanding soft tissue work, dynamic warm-ups, and assisted stretching because these areas will really make you stand out as a personal trainer. These three areas are typically skipped during a workout program, whereas they should really be the main focus as they can collectively provide more benefit than most workout programs.

The exercise program below, directly corresponds to the **Athletic** and **Balanced** exercise templates from the previous section. The main workout template below still works for most other client goals, however, you'll find some differences.

For example, the **Strength Gain** template doesn't focus on power exercises but will focus on exercise tempo and single-joint exercises. Additionally, the **Heart Health** and **Weight Loss** templates focus on full body strength routines and frequent endurance workouts. All goals and workouts have a different focus, and the workout below focuses on a client who wants to spend a little more time strengthening their entire body without the goal of being a bodybuilder. There's a lot to discuss, so let's dive in.

Exercise order can be a difficult concept to understand and also has much variation throughout the fitness industry. In my experience, the best method to use (for most client goals) is to perform power exercises first, then core (main, multi-joint muscles), and lastly assisted (single-joint) exercises.

I start with power exercises because it takes much mental focus and the body's power stores are the first energy system to be used during activity. Here are some of the best power exercises:

- Jumping in place (eg. jumping jacks, squat jump)
- Bounding (eg. skip)
- Throws (eg. chest pass)
- Depth jumps - advanced

- Power clean - advanced
- Power snatch - advanced
- Jump squat - advanced
- Push press - advanced

At this point, your clients will be mentally focused, their entire body will be warmed up, and most muscles will have a little fatigue. Next up are the core or multi-joint movements which typically involve larger muscle groups. Within a program, you want to make sure your clients are performing at least one of the following (preferably two) activities each week: knee dominant, hip dominant, horizontal press, vertical press, horizontal pull, vertical pull. Coaching this type of program will provide muscle balance and quickly help discover weaknesses. Here are a few exercises for the core (main) or multi-joint movements:

Knee dominant

- Back squat
- Front squat
- Single-leg squat

Hip dominant

- Back extension
- Deadlift
- Single leg deadlift

Horizontal press

- Bench press
- Push-up
- Cable fly

Vertical press

- Seated shoulder press
- Standing dumbbell press

Horizontal pull

- Bent over row
- Standing cable row

Vertical pull

- Chin-up
- Pull-up
- Lat pull down

Additionally, make sure you balance the number of opposing movements, which consist of the following: knee vs. hip dominant, horizontal push vs. pull, vertical push vs. pull. For example, most personal trainers and exercisers place a heavy focus on knee dominant and horizontal push exercises because they work on muscle groups that are on the front of the body and easily viewable. However, this often causes imbalances and injury.

The last part of your client's exercise program can be assisted or single-joint exercises. I'm including trunk (aka deep abs, core) exercises in single-joint exercises even though some exercises will be multi-joint. Here's a list of assisted exercises:

Trunk exercise

- Plank
- Stability ball rollouts
- Half-kneeling stability chop
- Landmine twists
- Swiss ball Russian twists

Other assisted exercises

- Bicep curls
- Triceps pull down

There are additional methods to select the exercise order that you may find beneficial. **Alternated** upper and lower body exercises are beneficial for untrained clients who have difficulty focusing on one body area at a time or if training times are limited. This method works well with circuit training and HIIT workouts. A similar method combines **push and pull** exercises to decrease movement fatigue. For example, a push movement could consist of a push-up and would be combined with a pull movement such as a standing row.

Two additional methods have a client perform two exercises together with little or no rest. A **compound** set has the client work the same muscle with two different exercises. And a **superset** has the client work opposite muscles (i.e. biceps, triceps) with two different exercises.

Another effective program for most beginner and intermediate clients is named Progressive Resistance Exercise (PRE) system and is comprised of the following: foam roll, dynamic warm-up, main workout with a set of light weights, main workout with a set of heavy weights, perform a third set of the main workout with the same weight from set two plus or minus 5-10 lbs., and then off to stretching. PRE is frequently used with athletes and untrained clients who want to develop strength quickly.

Stretching

After the main workout, it's best to end a training session with stretching. As with the warm-up, there are different types of stretching that can be used at the end of a session and I highly recommend assisted stretching if you have experience. Assisted stretching means that you're helping your client stretch by maneuvering their limbs and joints while they stay as passive as possible. It's much more effective than self-stretching because you're able to increase the client's flexibility with simple techniques. (If you're interested in learning more, I suggest researching PNF stretching.)

Many personal trainers choose to teach their client's self-stretching techniques, which can be used by the client with or without your oversight. No matter what stretching technique you employ, there are typical muscle groups that need to be stretched.

For most clients, the muscle groups that typically need to be stretched are as follows: neck, chest, lats, torso rotation, groin, hamstrings, quads, calves, hip flexors, and IT band. Again, you can find stretching instructions on YouTube and many other resources.

Each client is different and will enjoy certain stretches over others. Also, selecting muscles to stretch depends on the workout recently completed. For example, if your client just completed a leg workout, you'll want to focus more on stretching their legs and less on their upper body.

Additional notes

Training loads, exercise timing, and additional exercise details are outside the scope of this book. But here are a few additional notes based on my experience.

When writing your exercise programs, I recommend describing exercise intensities using light, moderate, and heavy naming conventions. Light intensity means the client can carry a conversation, moderate intensity means a client is having difficulty carrying a conversation, and heavy intensity means the client is unable to hold a conversation.

Another quick note, **periodization** takes a lot of focus to develop because most programs that utilize periodization are based on volume, load, and tempo. For most clients, spending much time on periodization is unnecessary (at first). Periodization works well once your client starts to gain experience with exercise technique. That being said, it's important to implement breaks into your training program. Typically a program will last 8 to 12 weeks and then the client should take a 7 to 10 day break to assist with mental and physical fatigue. The break should consist of fun workouts such as sport, dance, etc. After the break, the program can be updated with different exercises.

Endurance should be performed after strength as your body is able to cope with these types of exercises the longest (aerobic system kicks in last). Endurance exercise may not be a part of everyone's program, but it's beneficial to add light to moderate endurance training into most client programs.

In the client session outlined in a previous section, the main strength training program will last 20 – 40 minutes accounting for warmup and stretching in an hour session. Successful personal trainers quickly coach their clients on foam rolling, dynamic stretching, and static stretching to be performed without the personal trainer's oversight (before and after the session, respectively). This allows for the personal trainer and client to spend more time on the main workout, discussing nutrition or otherwise building value.

Each client will have a different strength training goal, and it can differ client by client and month by month. Exercise volume can be tied to a goal and usually follows this pattern (associated with core exercises previously explained):

- Power: 3 – 5 sets, 1 – 5 reps
- Strength: 2 – 6 sets, 1 – 6 reps
- Hypertrophy (muscle growth): 3 – 6 sets, 6 – 12 reps
- Endurance: 2 – 3 sets, 12 – 20 reps

There are many additional coaching ideas you will want to learn so that you can build immediate success. A few successful tips that can bridge your experience gap are the following:

- One of the most overlooked coaching cues is to remind your client to breathe during exercises. It seems silly but make this your top priority.
- Another top priority as a health coach is to prevent injuries in training. If your client has an injury in a training session, it's your fault.

- Flashy exercises may be good for some clients or your own workouts, but most clients do well with simple exercises.

- A good goal is to focus more on a client's technique than the number of reps and sets they perform. If a client's form looks bad after one set, you need to take a step back. Poor form leads to injuries, which leads to time off from training and less money for you.

- Skills-based training is performed at the beginning of a workout, such as sports skills (i.e. dribbling, juggling), agility and balance.

- Understand that volume, not weight, builds bulky muscles. If a client's goal is to build strength, it's beneficial to use heavier weights. You'll get initial push back more often from female clients because there's a big myth that heavy weight means bigger muscles – you'll need to educate these clients.

- Confirm that the exercise set times can fit inside your daily program session. Too many exercises that take a long time to perform can kill a workout plan.

- Write exercise programs that have the client move in all anatomical planes – sagittal, frontal, transverse.

Building a full meal program

Meal programs will also differ in many aspects including frequency, volume, and composition. I'll describe the basics of all meal programs and dive into specific diet types.

The goal of this section is to give you the basic tools to create your own meal programs. If an idea or tool isn't familiar to you, please do further research to expand your understanding.

Let's get started.

As a general overview, here are the basics of a meal program:

- Consume 3 – 5 meals per day (full meals or snacks)
- Each meal should have a balance of protein, fats, and carbs
- Drink plenty of water
- Intake minimal amounts of processed foods (i.e. sugars, meats)
- Avoid consuming too much cholesterol and many "bad" fats

It's important to understand that each meal program will have a balance of protein, fats, and carbs (macronutrients) – no program can be sustained without focusing on all three components. Most meals should consist of a mix of protein, fats, and carbs in a balance consistent with your diet type. It's best to start with the meal template (i.e. weight gain) that best matches your client's goal, find the "What to eat" section, and select foods that will provide a macronutrient balance.

As a client transitions into their new diet, one of the hardest parts will be consistency, so make sure you're empathetic to their changing lifestyles. Additionally, clients will have individual reactions to different diets and not every diet will work for each person – you'll have to make adjustments to the meal plan.

It's difficult to lock down rules around all diet types so I'll relate meal planning back to a previous section. Below, I detail the foods typical of the meal plan templates previously discussed – weight gain, low carb, gluten-free, paleo, vegan, Mediterranean.

Weight gain diet

Weight gain is a goal for people who want to gain mass, which is typical of athletes, bodybuilders, and clients with a smaller frame. A weight gain diet is comprised of the following:

What to eat

- Meats such as lean ground beef, chicken breast, tilapia

- Dairy such as cottage cheese, milk, Greek yogurt
- Grains
- Nuts and seeds such as almonds, walnuts, quinoa
- Fruits such as oranges, cantaloupe, apples
- Potatoes
- Eggs
- "Good" fats
- Cereal
- Rice
- Pasta
- Vegetables such as beets, spinach

What to avoid

- "Bad" or too many fats
- Heavily processed food
- Added sugars

Additional notes

- Some fat will come along with the weight gain (even if you're gaining a lot of muscle with exercise)
- Eat three meals a day, plus a snack before and after a workout
- Eat more during meals, eat more meals, eat calorie dense foods, eat more protein, consume liquids with high amounts of calories for easier digestion, track calories
- A typical weight gain program, increases caloric intake by 500 – 1000 calories/day

Low carb diet

Low carb diets are for people who want to decrease their carb intake, which is typical of clients who want to lose weight and decrease their likelihood of diseases. A low carb diet is comprised of the following:

What to eat

- Meat such as beef, pork, lamb and poultry
- Fish such as salmon, sardines, herring
- Seafood
- Eggs
- Natural fat and high-fat sauces such as butter, hollandaise sauce, coconut oil
- Vegetables that grow above the ground such as cauliflower, broccoli, Brussel sprouts, bok choy, zucchini, olives, onions, peppers
- Dairy products such as butter (natural, full-fat), cream, sour cream
- Nuts and seeds
- Berries
- Non-gluten grains

What to avoid

- Sugars such as soft drinks, candy, chocolate, pastries, ice cream
- Starch such as bread, pasta, rice, potatoes
- Gluten grains
- Trans fats
- Artificial sweeteners
- Processed foods
- High Omega-6 seeds and vegetable oils
- "Diet" and "low fat" products
- Margarine
- Beer

Additional notes

- Typical macronutrient combination of 5% carbs, 35% protein, 65% fats

- Typically consume under 50g of carbohydrates/day

Gluten-free diet

Gluten-free diets are for people who need to eliminate gluten in their diets typically because of gluten sensitivity or celiac disease. A gluten-free diet is comprised of the following:

What to eat

- Corn in all forms such as corn flour, cornmeal, grits
- Plain rice in all forms such as white, brown, wild, basmati
- Nuts and nut butters
- Beans
- Coconut
- Quinoa
- Flax
- Millet
- Soy
- Tapioca
- Arrowroot
- Milk products such as butter, real cheese, plain yogurt, most ice cream
- Vegetable oils
- Plain fruit
- Vegetables
- Meat
- Seafood
- Potatoes
- Healthy fats
- Dark chocolate
- Eggs
- Legumes
- Spices

- Distilled alcohol

What not to eat

- Wheat in all forms such as spelt, Kamut, durum, semolina, cake flour, couscous
- Barley
- Malt
- Rye
- Breaded meat
- Licorice

Additional notes

- Typical foods with these ingredients are bread, pasta, cereal, beer, cakes, pie, pastries, cookies, crackers, biscuits, sauces, dressings, gravies, soy sauce
- Read all food labels and restaurant menus

Paleo diet

Paleo diets are for people who want to mimic our hunter-gather ancestors and eat more natural foods. The paleo diet is comprised of the following:

What to eat

- Meat such as skinless turkey breast, lean pork tenderloin, sirloin beef steak, skinless chicken breast
- Fish such as shrimp, halibut, broiled tuna
- Eggs
- Vegetables such as artichoke, asparagus, broccoli, cauliflower, carrots, celery, eggplant, kale, lettuce, onions, peppers, pumpkin, seaweed
- Fruit such as bananas, blueberries, boysenberries, cherries, figs, grapefruit, grapes, kiwi, lemon, orange, pineapple, watermelon

- Nuts and seeds such as almonds, cashews, hazelnuts, macadamia nuts, pecans, pumpkin seeds, walnuts
- Herbs and spices
- Healthy fats
- Oils

What not to eat

- Most dairy
- Processed meats such as ham lunch meat, dry salami
- Cereals
- Legumes
- Refined sugar
- High fat - low protein ratio foods such as T-bone steak, lamb shoulder roast, eggs, beef ribs, link pork sausage, bacon, hot dog, ground beef.
- Processed foods such as sugar, high fructose corn syrup, grains, artificial sweeteners,
- Margarine

Additional notes

- A typical meal consists of tons of vegetables, serving of lean protein, healthy fat (eg. coconut oil)
- Eat as much lean meats, fish, and seafood as possible
- Eat as much fruits and non-starchy veggies as possible
- Eat until full
- Calorie counting is not encouraged
- Consider supplementing vitamin D and probiotics
- Doesn't really focus on a macronutrient breakdown, however, an estimate is close to 22 – 40% carbs, 19 – 35% protein, 28 – 58% fats

Vegan diet

Vegan diets are for people who want to eliminate animal products in their diets. The vegan diet is comprised of the following:

What to eat

- Fruit such as apples, oranges, berries, pineapples, grapes
- Vegetables such as asparagus, kale, broccoli, celery, spinach
- Nuts and seeds such as almonds, cashews, peanut butter
- Carbs such as potatoes, pasta, bread
- Beans and legumes such as tofu, edamame, hummus, chickpeas
- Non-dairy milk such as coconut, almond, soy, hemp
- Chocolate such as dark, soy, made from rice milk
- Meat alternatives such as tempeh, seitan, jackfruit, mushrooms, lentils, textured vegetable protein, gluten-free vegan meat
- Dairy alternatives such as coconut ice cream, almond yogurt, vegan cheese
- Leafy greens such as kale, swiss chard, collard greens, spinach
- Whole grains such as quinoa, millet, barley, buckwheat

What not to eat

- Meat
- Poultry
- Fish and seafood
- Dairy
- Eggs
- Bee products
- Animal-based ingredients

Additional notes

- Typical sources of protein include: lentils, chickpeas, tofu, peanut butter, soy milk, almonds, spinach, rice, whole wheat bread, broccoli, kale
- May need to supplement diet with a B12 vitamin, iron, vitamin D
- Be careful with the amount of soy consumed

Mediterranean diet

Mediterranean diets are for people who want to eat a healthier diet overall without eliminating many common foods. The Mediterranean diet is comprised of the following:

What to eat

- Fruits such as apples, bananas, grapes, dates, figs
- Vegetables such as broccoli, kale, spinach, onions, carrots, cucumbers
- Whole grains such as brown rice, barley, corn, pasta
- Legumes such as beans, peas, lentils, peanuts
- Nuts and seeds such as almonds, walnuts, macadamia nuts, cashews
- Olive oil and canola oil
- Herbs and spices such as garlic, basil, mint, rosemary
- Fish and seafood such as salmon, trout, tuna, oysters, clams, mussels
- Tubers such as potatoes, turnips, yams

Eat in moderation

- Poultry such as chicken, duck, turkey
- Eggs
- Dairy such as cheese, yogurt
- Red wine

- Red meat (rare)

What to avoid

- Butter
- Salt
- Added sugars
- Processed meat and foods
- Refined grains
- Refined oil

Additional Notes

- Fish is the main source of animal protein as it is a good source of lean meat

First client session

An hour before the first session, confirm that your client is still able to attend the appointment; this is usually accomplished by a quick mobile text message. Gather all your materials, including the client meal program, exercise program, Client Session Sign-in Sheet, and essential pieces of equipment.

Fifteen minutes before your session, make sure you're dressed appropriately using my previous recommendations, including: branded t-shirt, exercise clothing, and athletic shoes. Confirm you also have all the necessary non-exercise equipment to keep the training session running smoothly.

Two minutes before the session, arrive at the designated meeting location and gather your energy. Be yourself, stay focused, and be prepared to connect with your client. When your client arrives, greet them and request their signature on the Client Session Sign-in Sheet. Afterwards, make your way to the fitness area while asking your client how they're feeling and then provide an overview of the upcoming training session.

It's important to follow the workout program as closely as possible, depending on the client's energy level. Throughout each activity, talk with your client to determine their comfort level. Take note of your client's movements, how they feel, and if they're struggling. It's important to communicate regularly so you can make the appropriate adjustments.

On the first session, you will want to end 10 – 15 minutes early so that you have time to discuss the overall health program. With all subsequent sessions, end 5 minutes early so that you can prepare for your next client. Additionally, if you haven't already set a regular training schedule, set a routine with your client. Having a regular workout schedule will help achieve your client's goals faster.

BUSINESS ADMINISTRATION

To sell to your first clients, make sure you have your Direct Debit paperwork and an Invoice ready. Be aware that direct debits may take a few days to set up between your client's bank and your business bank.

Additionally, it's good practice to keep a physical and/or digital copy of all client records in case you need them down the road (eg. legal issues). You should keep a copy of all Client Intake Forms, meal and exercise programs, Client Sign-in Sheets, all training notes, and invoices.

BONUS: The importance of communication

You need to be able to balance the different personality types, with clients ranging from chatty to silent. When I first started personal training, chatty clients would run my training sessions and hour-long workouts would honestly result in only 10 minutes of exercises. I also experienced clients who wouldn't say more than two words during our sessions, and it was very difficult to understand their comfort level in our program.

But why did I care? I was getting paid, so wasn't that enough? Enough wasn't good enough for me. I realized I wasn't providing value to my clients, which in turn was reducing my sales in the long term.

I changed my mindset from letting clients determine session communication to leading conversations. I focused on verbal and nonverbal communication cues and made it clear to each of my clients the benefits of regular discussion, such as faster goal attainment, more comfort during workouts, and having fun.

Leading communication means you have to focus on the client throughout the entire workout, not just while they're performing exercises. Listen to what your client is saying, watch how their body is reacting, and use verbal and nonverbal communication cues to understand what your client needs at any given time.

Excellent communication is an overlooked "soft" skill that can turn a mediocre personal trainer into a successful one. Throughout the training session, you should ask your clients questions such as, "How is this exercise working for you today?", "How are you feeling?", "How is your day?", "Did you get enough sleep last night?"

Your ability to direct conversation and extract important health information further extends to building a relationship with your client, which builds value and leads to more sales. Directing conversation means you need to understand your client's personality and what they care about (their priorities).

Chatty clients are more prevalent than extremely quiet ones, which is why I'll focus on leading conversations with chatty clients. If you have a client who cares deeply about their finances and is also so chatty that you're unable to complete a full session, you can say, "I don't want to waste your money because we're not hitting your fitness goals. I want to make sure we're meeting our objectives today and every day. It's beneficial if we work hard during the exercise and then we can chat during your breaks."

For another example, if you have a chatty client you can say, "I enjoy chatting and getting to know you, I just want to make sure you understand that if we continue chatting this much we may not reach your original fitness goals. We can chat and exercise or we just need to readjust your program and goals."

You need to have the flexibility in your personality to work with different personality and communication types. You also need to be flexible in the way you communicate with the different personality types and their daily energy levels.

I want to remind you that each client and each session is different. If a client is having a hard day, it's probably okay that fitness activities are a lower priority and you provide empathy through emotional support. Missing one day of exercise isn't going to destroy a fitness program.

Activity: *Write two conversations, directing a chatty and quiet client on the importance of regular communication.*

Full-service Personal Training

What's full-service personal training? Full-service personal training is your key to success. It means increasing value for you, by increasing value for your clients and prospects. Full-service personal training is anticipating and providing your clients' and prospects' needs before they communicate them.

Part of full-service training is to deliver services when your client isn't physically meeting with you, providing items such as a food journal, sleep journal, or fitness program. When the client is with you, your full-service personal training might include activities such as carrying comfort items (i.e. Kleenex, hair ties), providing emotional comfort, writing a fun exercise session that involves playing their favorite sport, and more.

With full-service personal training, you treat every person you meet as a prospect, you treat every prospect like a client, and you treat your clients like family. Full- service personal training is about creating value for your brand. Increase your value, and you increase your price tag.

Activity: *Record activities that will turn you into a full-service personal trainer.*

SALES AND MARKETING

Marketing

Marketing is everything a company does to acquire customers. Up until this point, I've given you marketing tools and reviewed how to apply the tools to gain success. To earn your first few clients, you'll need to continue your marketing efforts by brainstorming ideas to acquire clients (or prospects).

There are many ways to market to, and gain, your first few clients. To help kick-off your brainstorming and marketing efforts, I'm providing a few marketing ideas below:

- Offer discounted or free sessions – these can be full length (60 minutes) or mini (30 minutes) sessions
- Host a fitness or health challenge with a prize. For example, market a 2-week step challenge with a prize for

1st ($100), 2nd ($75), and 3rd ($50). You'll receive every participant's contact information, which gives you the opportunity to discuss your personal training services with them

- Create a 6 – 8 week program and offer it to a specific group or business. For example, offer a program to decrease blood pressure to people with heart issues – additionally, you can reach out to hospitals as they'll have a pool of prospects

Activity: *Make a list of* at least *three marketing ideas to help acquire your first clients.*

Sales

Delivering a sales pitch is not a talent or an inborn gift. Pitching, like anything else, is a skill. No matter how difficult a skill seems, it can always be learned depending on your determination. In this section, we review one of the greatest challenges to an unsuccessful personal trainer — the sales pitch.

In earlier chapters, I recommended using every opportunity to speak with people about your business and gain prospects. The goal isn't to just gain a prospect, but to gain a client by selling your services.

It's beneficial to understand that people have a vision for success and it's your job to help them honestly realize that vision. It's also beneficial to not take objection personally. Just because somebody doesn't purchase your services, it doesn't mean anything negative about you as a person. Stay confident, perfect your sales technique, and find a way to match a prospect's vision to your offered value.

Pitch tools

You benefit by coming prepared to your pitch with specific client information, and the best tools to bring with you are the following:

1. Basic meal plan
2. Basic exercise plan
3. Price sheet
4. Food journal
5. Initial consultation forms
6. Notes from physical assessment

How to sell

There are numerous selling methods and many of them have merit. An effective method that I highlight below is the STRONG method, which simplifies the sales pitch into key steps. Using this method, you will have 10 – 15 minutes to make your pitch at the end of the fitness assessment. The STRONG method is separated into a short introduction (3 minutes), an explanation of what makes you so great (5 - 10 minutes), and time to offer the deal using emotional connection (2 minutes).

After the physical assessment, it's important to find an area where you can speak to the prospect alone, which will help build a personal connection. Below, we dive into the STRONG method.

<u>S</u>et the framework: You are leading the pitch and it's up to you to set the tone. One tone that works well in sales is to put a time limit on the meeting such as, "We only have 15 minutes to finish." This keeps the prospect focused on what you're about to say.

Also, you want to provide background on the problem and your track record for success. For example, "I've worked with clients that had a similar background to you, and we were able to achieve their goals within six months using my methods."

<u>T</u>ell the story: One of your greatest obstacles in closing a sale is your client losing focus because they anticipate your speech and offer. The answer is to grab their attention with a story, to make the pitch more personal and attention-grabbing. For example, "A former client lost 5% body fat over an eight month period with my guidance and hard work."

Reveal the intrigue: You need to grab your prospect's attention every few minutes and you can do this by creating tension with focused risk, danger, uncertainty, and time constraints. For example, "You were unable to meet your health goals on your own and I only see you achieving your goals with a coach who can start with you immediately. If you wait any longer, your goals will become harder and harder to achieve."

Offer the prize: This is where you get to show your value! Use all the necessary tools (i.e. basic exercise program, S.M.A.R.T. goals) to show your value such as, "I create an individual health plan for short and long-term goals, so there is never a question of where you are or where your training is heading."

Nail the hook point: Most financial decisions are not made with logic but with emotion. You need to get your prospect fully emotionally engaged. For example, "There's a possibility we may not be a good fit for each other. However, if we do partner together, I believe we can meet your health goals quickly."

Get the deal. The last part of the pitch is the most critical. Most personal trainers are unsuccessful sales closers and act "needy" at this point which changes the framework from the prospect needing your value to you needing their value (money). You can avoid these pitfalls by adding a limited purchasing time into your pitch such as, "I have two more minutes until I meet with my next potential client."

Using the STRONG method for sales pitches, I created a simple sales pitch example (below) designed for a prospect that has a goal of weight loss.

Example pitch

This part is going to be short as I only have 10 minutes until my next appointment.

I've worked with dozens of clients with similar goals and baseline levels. One client, Jerry, followed my instructions, and we had a great partnership. Over a two year period, he reduced his weight, body fat, blood pressure and heart rate. Once he took his life into his own hands and decided to partner with me, he was able to focus until he achieved his goals. Jerry went from being clinically obese to a healthy BMI and body fat percent.

You came to these training sessions because you were motivated to change your health. In my experience, motivation is a great starting point but it cannot achieve goals by itself. Your motivation needs to quickly be partnered with focused activities. Personal training partners your motivation with a specific program to meet your health goals.

Your old habits aren't working. In your own words, your health is at a low point and it needs to change — immediately. We need to shift your old habits into healthy habits, and we need to use your current motivation immediately before you lose focus.

My personal training services are for overweight clients who are dissatisfied with their health, their current habits and haven't been able to meet their goals. My services create an individual health plan, which tailors each program, workout, and exercise to fit your needs. I build on your current motivation and focus your workouts to achieve positive health. Unlike other programs with a one-size-fits-all approach, I work with you every day through one-on-one training, exercise homework, meal plans, and health tips.

[This is where I review the basic meal and exercise plan and how they will accomplish the client's goals.]

Clients that work with me often see results much faster than with other personal trainers and programs. They often drop weight or clothing sizes within a few weeks.

In my experience, my connection to my clients is my highest value, and it's what keeps us both motivated to achieve your goals. However, there's a real possibility we might not be right for each other.

(This is where I pause to let the information sink in)

But, if this partnership works out, I can tell we could combine to exceed your goals.

Most clients and programs fail because there's a lack of communication, accountability, structure, and respect. I'm selective about my clients because I get committed to them and their goals. What other programs lack, I provide in full.

I communicate with my clients every few days to review their health and this helps keep my clients accountable. I provide a structured meal and exercise plan while my clients are with me and at home. And I gain respect by giving respect. I'm not late to our sessions and if I need to reschedule for any reason, I give advanced warning. I care too much about my clients to see them fail. It's why I'm so selective about the clients I take on.

Over these last two days of assessments, I've learned a lot about you. I think I can guide you to your goals and we could have a great partnership. I have a few spots open in my schedule for a new committed client that will most likely fill up this week if you don't fill it.

I have two more minutes until I need to leave for my next potential client.

(This is where I pause and wait for the prospect's response)

Pitch downfall

One of the worst things you can do in a pitch is to show your neediness for the sale. You will fail if you ask for a sale using sentences such as, "Do you still think it's a good deal?", "So what do you think?", or "We can sign a deal right away if you want us to." These sentences put too much power into the hands of your prospect.

Even if you desperately need the sale, do not act like it when you're speaking to your prospect. Focus on the conversation around your value, what you offer your clients, and how you're much better than all other options including other personal trainers or people exercising on their own.

Additionally, as you see in the pitch example, a simple way to reduce sounding needy is to input a time limit, "I have two more minutes until I need to leave for my next potential client" because it shows you're leading the conversation and your time is valuable.

Activity: *With respect to your niche and target client, write a pitch outline.*

Pitch success

A sales pitch can be difficult for many personal trainers, but there are a few ways for you to quickly gain experience. Practice, practice, practice.

As with all skills, intentional practice builds any skill and pitching works the same way. Practice your sales pitch (preceding activity) to gain confidence and experience. Just as important, remember the value you bring to people's lives. You are worth the money your clients are spending on their health. Take confidence in the value you offer.

Objection handling

You've just pitched a prospect, describing all the value you can bring to their life, but the prospect still objects to the sale. There are two ways to deal with prospect's objections: address them or don't.

In the pitch example, I use time as a critical factor in the prospect making an emotional decision for the sale. If you want to use time to your advantage and the prospect objects, you can simply state that you don't currently have time to address their questions, and suggest they can reach out when they're committed to their goals. Heads up, this method will not work with everyone.

If you choose to answer the prospect's objections, how do you move forward successfully? With each objection, there is a specific path to success, which I highlight below.

Step 1 – Gratitude: Thank the prospect for giving you an opportunity to address their objections. If a prospect is objecting they aren't saying no; they're giving you the opportunity to have them say yes. Ask about all their objections up front so you can address them all at once.

Step 2 – Empathy: As I've discussed throughout this book, empathy is one of the strongest characteristics of a successful personal trainer. To show your empathy, you can start by saying, "I'm sorry you feel that way", "I hear what you're saying", or "I sometimes hear similar objections." Empathy helps diffuse tension.

Step 3 – Discover: Find out what's really going on by asking open-ended questions. If the prospect is able to answer with a "yes" or a "no," then you've phrased the questions incorrectly. If you find the conversation stalling, start asking "why?" to drill down to the real reasons behind an objection. (The "Why" Method is used throughout the business world to discover client values).

Step 4 – Ask, probe, confirm: Continue to ask questions and ask prospects to clarify if something needs further attention. Your goal is open communication, discover the issues, and provide value. You also want to review the prospects discussion points in your own words.

Step 5 – Show value: Throughout the conversation, you will have identified the prospect's pain points, such as how their health affects their life, social interactions, self-perception, etc. Pain can cost a person financially, psychologically, and emotionally. By defining a prospect's pain points, you're able to specifically define the prospect's fears and needs, and discuss how you're able to solve them.

Step 6 – Proof and customer references: If possible, back up your value claims with client anecdotes and references. Objections are much easier to handle if you have proof of previous success. It provides a tangible connection from the prospect's needs to your value.

Let's review the most common prospect objections and how to handle them by addressing pain points. Additionally, keep in mind that price is not the real issue behind an objection; it's a matter of an individual's priority and values.

No time – Time issues all depend on life priorities. Having success with health influences all other areas of a prospect's life. For example, is financial or professional success important to the prospect? If the prospect is physically healthier, they'll be able to work more effectively while at work. The prospect will be able to have more energy, passion, and happiness for the things they're doing. Over the last two meetings, you may have picked up on activities that can be deprioritized, such as watching television, which you can use to your advantage. If the prospect decreased watching television from 90 minutes to 30 minutes a day, they could have enough time for both activities. If you suggest a reprioritization of their daily life, they can have time to be healthy. You need to deliver health goals as "must-haves" instead of "nice-to-haves."

It's too expensive – You can ask further questions such as, "What price do you put on your health? What price do you put on your fitness? What price do you put on achieving your goals?" Discuss the prospect's current health level, any issues they're having and the outcomes (i.e. more energy, less stress) that your training program will deliver. If a prospect tries to workout on their own, they'll waste much time and energy developing a program that is only fractionally successful in comparison to yours. The cost doesn't matter because you're delivering so much value that the prospect isn't able to see success with their goals without thinking of you.

I have to think about it – You can probe further such as, "What do you have to think about?" Dive into the prospect's responses. Remember, the prospect has a stronger connection to you and your value while they are in front of you. If they leave you without purchasing, it allows doubts to flood their mind. You're trying to break their old patterns, which is why they initially came to see you. Their old patterns haven't been working, or haven't been working well enough to reach their goals.

I have to ask my partner – Gently ask the prospect, "What do you need to ask your partner about? Each individual person has their own aspirations and needs. You have goals that overlap with your partner in your relationship, but the goals we've discussed together are specific to your needs." If the prospect lives a healthier life, they can give their partner more energy, more time, more focus, more passion, and more attention. Another successful idea is to request that the partner joins your sessions and all three of you can train together, which would provide the following benefits to the prospect: save money (per person), provide more time to connect, and increase health. On your end, you get two clients as opposed to the one or possibly zero clients if the prospect doesn't purchase your services.

I have a previous injury – If a prospect has an injury, it should be a welcome objection to hear because you can help alleviate pain through massage, stretching, strengthening, and the training sessions can be a recurrent source of motivation. *Note:* you should work with their health provider (physician, physical therapist) to make a health action plan.

I've never had a personal trainer – This objection should be one of the easier ones to handle because you're presenting so much new value to the prospect. If they've never worked out at all and they don't adopt your services, it may take months to fully realize how much time and effort working with you can save them. If the prospect has previously exercised, then they can understand how much effort it takes to create health programs and will appreciate the knowledge, focus, and motivation you can provide.

Know-it-all attitudes – Your first instinct may be to push back or give a prospect the same attitude. Remember you're here to help get them to their goals. If the prospect knew everything, they wouldn't have met with you or they would already be at their goals. Moreover, everybody should have a personal trainer — personal trainers should have personal trainers. In reality, even elite athletes have trainers who guide them on a daily basis. Even if a prospect understands exercise form, program creation, and goal management, it's impossible for them to provide the same amount of focus and motivation to match a successful personal trainer. You provide more value than an individual can reproduce for themselves, including motivation, inspiration, program variation, intuiting a client's needs when they aren't fully communicating, and more.

Activity: *Using the list of objections, select one and write out a complete transcript example where you answer their objections using the success path (steps 1 – 6). Bonus points for writing a transcript for all the aforementioned objections and for practicing objection conversations with a friend or coworker.*

LOOK BACK TO MOVE FORWARD

Sometimes, the best the way to move forward is to look to the past!

This cliché couldn't be truer than right now. If you're an experienced personal trainer and realize your sales need to be better, it's time to look to your past.

Review your old prospect and client notes to identify the lost opportunities. Ask yourself questions such as, "Why didn't this prospect purchase from me?", "What excuses did they give me?", "What objections couldn't I handle?", "Why didn't a client renew their personal training sessions?" Identifying answers to these questions will give you insight into the areas of your business that need improvement.

From your review, you may start to notice a theme: a pattern of why and when you couldn't complete a sale. If you find a pattern, great! You just identified a negative habit in yourself, which is the hardest part of changing who you are. Now you can work on correcting that previous deficiency.

Activity: *If you're an experienced personal trainer, review your lost opportunities from the past 1, 3, 6, or 12 months. If possible, identify negative patterns and plan how you will change that habit in the future using the outlined pitch and objection handling techniques.*

This last chapter has been filled with information. I encourage you to go back and refer to it often as you apply the principles and knowledge in your personal training and your business. I don't expect you to memorize all of these tools, so keep this book close to continuously build on your successes or to help you out of failures. Keep persevering and don't give up.

Chapter Eight

Keep Your Momentum

"There are no secrets to success. It's the result of preparation, hard work and learning from failure."
- Colin Powell-

Hey, Luke! Great post on Ted's Facebook page about compassion for your clients.

I found it really inspiring. What are your plans?

John, the business exec, was asking after you the other day.

He is looking for a lifestyle coach to help him.

He is needing a bit more in depth help with his diet and his busy lifestyle.

Can I give him your contact details?

I would love to chat sometime about your future plans.

Give me a call.

Kirsten

Kirsten's message had just popped up on Luke's Facebook page. He had started writing for Ted and promoting his soon-to-be new business as a personal trainer and lifestyle coach. Ted had encouraged him to study further and Luke was working on becoming a qualified lifestyle coach. His plan was to keep working with Ted part-time, but was also aiming to become an independent personal trainer in a month or two. Ted had offered Luke a space in his gym for rent so that he could work with his personal clients, and Luke was slowly finding the courage to step into being an independent personal trainer.

Ted walked into the office, he was moving about now without crutches. Luke couldn't believe it was the same guy that had been hobbling six months ago. Ted had been diligent in applying all the rehab exercises prescribed by his physical therapist (and exercises from his own experience) and the strength and improvement was evident to all who came to the gym.

Ted's journey to recovery had not been an easy one. When he first started to walk without crutches, he had lost his balance and fallen a few times — but he'd kept at it, learned from the mistake and tried again. He regularly tested his strength and ability and tweaked his program according to his progress.

"Ted, your rehab has been phenomenal. You look like a completely different guy!"

"I could say the same to you, Luke," Ted smiled, "You've inspired me with your courage and determination to apply all the steps and advice that I've given you. You look, and are, completely different to when you first walked in here." As he said that, he stumbled a little, but caught himself. His legs were a bit tired from working with Peter. Ted continued, "That stumble reminds me. I've given you so much information, but there's one piece of advice that I think you can *now* handle – fail, and fail fast."

Luke was shocked to hear this. *Fail?* That's the opposite of success, right? He was stunned by Ted's words. Ted followed up by saying, "You're never going to create a perfect program; you're never going to create a perfect business. What you want to do is take your ideas and test them immediately. Gather your exercises and programs and try them out. Do the same with your business ideas. And do it quickly. Most of the time these things will fail. It's the successful personal trainer; the successful person, who can pick themselves up quickly, learn from their failures and move towards success. If you have success with a client, ask for a referral, ask for the testimonials, and use them to help with sales and marketing. But if you fail, learn from those mistakes. Talk to the client, to your business partners when you have them and, when you have your gym, talk to your employees and ask them what you can do better next time; discover how you failed — and fix it."

Failure was something that Luke had never seen as a good thing before he started working with Ted. Many of their clients came to the gym with the fear of failure and Ted had graciously helped them change their attitude towards it. Each time they made mistakes, failed in workouts or had "bad diet days," he encouraged them to look at their mistakes, to learn from them, and to move on. Ted, always going the extra mile, helped each client apply that principle in their lives, in their families and in their careers. As Luke reflected on this, he found the courage to take the next step in his career...

Hey Kirsten, good to hear from you.

Thanks for reaching out to me.

I am doing so well, thanks for referring me to Ted.

It will be great to catch up. Please do give my details to John.

I'm working as an independent personal trainer and I'd love to help him.

Chat soon.

Luke

> "You build on failure. You use it as a stepping stone.
> Close the door on the past. You don't try to forget the
> mistakes, but you don't dwell on it. You don't let it have
> any of your energy, or any of your time, or any of your
> space."
> - Johnny Cash-

So, you have your first clients, now what? To keep the momentum, do not get comfortable with your business. Successful businesses have a grow-or-die mentality. There are many personal trainers who are competing for the same pool of clients and hundreds more will set up their business over your career. It's your job to stay on top of your success or suffer the consequences.

Every personal trainer has the opportunity to be successful, but it's much easier to maintain success than it is to acquire it.

Losing a client

So you've just lost a client? Uh-oh, that hurts. Over the years, I've personally lost many clients for a range of reasons. Understand that clients canceling is an experience that every business deals with; it's normal and natural for clients to move in and out of your life, like any other relationship. It's nothing to fret over.

Take this loss as a learning opportunity. Grow from this experience so it doesn't happen again. If you don't grow, your brand will suffer. Use failures as an opportunity for growth. Ask yourself what you can do better next time so that you don't experience loss. If you do not grow, you will *not* reach your full potential and you will not reach your full potential without continuous growth.

Iterate and win

Ever wonder how software companies are able to grow exponentially? Amongst many things, iteration is at the forefront of their success. Iteration is the process of repetitive improvement, and that's your secret weapon for success, especially in the fitness industry where progress is very slow.

Understand your failures and successes so that you can iterate on your business processes. To provide more detail, software companies use a process called the development life cycle to improve their products. Google, Facebook, Airbnb and Uber didn't become amazing products overnight; they released a product and kept iterating as their users (that's us) changed their wants and needs. The process of a development life cycle is described with the following activities — design, implement, test, improve.

To succeed, I'm adapting the software development life cycle to the personal training business so that you can achieve similar high growth. Using the same life cycle activities, you will apply the development life cycle to each facet (i.e. marketing, sales etc.) of your personal training business. For each part of your business you will perform the following: design (completed in the Tools section), implement (completed in the Integrating Tools section), test, and improve.

If you're an experienced personal trainer, you have already tested your product (services) and can improve them by reviewing what's worked and what hasn't worked (luckily you reviewed lost opportunities in the Book First Clients section).

If you're a new personal trainer, you'll have to test and improve your services on a rolling basis. The iterative development life cycle is a constant activity, which means your job is *never* done. Remember that you can always improve your services in one way or another.

Last point on iteration that is renowned in the software world – fail quickly. Failing quickly is a sign of pride in the software world. Get this, Google would rather hire people who've failed many times and then achieved success over people who've only experienced success. Why? Because knowing how to cope with failure is a key to success.

Successful personal trainers didn't achieve greatness without doing poorly and failing along the way. And neither will you. Don't be careful; race towards failure. The faster you fail, the faster you'll be on your way towards success. Make it a point to fail faster than the personal trainer next to you.

Fail to succeed

Measure everything

Additionally, you can find out how your services are working by analyzing business metrics such as tracking the number of leads acquired, conversions from leads into prospects (the first session), conversions from the first session into the second session, and conversions from prospect to client. You should also get subjective feedback from your clients such as how they feel about your program design, session flow, communication, and connection.

It's beneficial to test everything. From the success of your business flyer to your logo, the exercises you choose, to the number of leads you bring in each month. If you can measure it (objectively or subjectively), you can improve it.

To analyze business metrics (i.e. the number of prospects converted to clients), you need to measure everything. This is why you take detailed notes during a fitness session, this is why we regularly assess clients, and why we keep track of all business, sales and marketing information – so it can be improved upon.

With detailed notes, you're able to understand the gaps in your business. Most personal trainers will spend years in a failing business because they only focus on the end results, sales. But when you measure everything, you're able to dig into the root cause of your sales issue, which may lead you to focus on a bad conversion from the first prospect assessment to the second.

In a measure-everything mindset, your failures are caught immediately and then you get the opportunity to improve your business. When you measure everything, you have objective facts that assist your sales pitch and it's easier to have honest conversations about what is, and isn't, working for your business.

Growth

How do you continue your success and extend it to adding clients 2, 3, 4,... 30?

Simplicity is key

I've given you mountains of information. It may seem like a lot and it is! So how do you simplify this knowledge to effectively create growth? Follow this simple four step process: get a client, make them happy, ask for a referral, and restart the cycle.

Continue this cycle until you're happy with your business, and soon enough you won't have to ask for referrals in order to get clients; prospects will come to you! In previous sections, you learned how to get a client, so now you'll learn how to make them happy.

Make your client happy

You need to take the first clients you've acquired and make sure they're happy – this is also known as client management. Client happiness increases your value and increases the number of referrals and testimonials you receive. Part of keeping your clients happy is to make sure they're doing okay with their programs and that they still enjoy your services (described in an earlier section).

It's beneficial to continuously test your clients by taking daily notes and regularly assessing their states of health. Continuously test physical measurements, BMI, strength, flexibility, endurance, nutrition and so on. Client management means providing continuous value and in return, you'll receive continuous payment for your efforts.

Now your business is firing on all cylinders. You're a full-service personal trainer, you write excellent fitness and diet programs, and your clients love you. What more can you give? Another good business practice is to reward your clients for their commitment by giving gifts. If they've been with you for six months or a year say thank you in some way, and they'll be extremely appreciative.

Gifts can come in many shapes and sizes such as reducing the price for a session or bundle, delivering health conscious gift cards (i.e. salad-based restaurant), or creating a before and after framed photo.

Gift giving is a frequent occurrence in the fitness industry. Most successful personal trainers provide gifts to their clients and often time's clients reciprocate with a gift of their own (financial or otherwise) or by zealously repurchasing your services. Rewarding with gifts increases the bond with your clients and increases your value.

Asking for the referral

In earlier parts of this book, I discussed how beneficial referrals are to gaining new business. Referrals can come from any source including family, friends, coworkers, neighbors, prospects, clients and from a successful brand. I also reviewed the benefits of referrals including lead generation, lower marketing costs, improved conversion rate and an increase in engagement.

I reviewed the Client Referral Form as one form of requesting a referral, but how else can you get a referral?

The first route is through a warm referral request. A warm referral is when you request a referral from people you've worked with in the past (prospect or client). After a few training sessions with a client, it's easy to request a referral verbally. I recommend that you speak to a specific goal you have been working towards and are on your way to achieving. Additionally, talk about your passion for the fitness industry and how you enjoy helping people. For example, when chatting with your client you can say:

"Our last three workouts have been great. You've increased your pull-up strength by 10 lbs., as well as your hamstring flexibility. I really enjoy helping people hit their goals and would appreciate the opportunity to help more people. Do you have any friends, family, or coworkers that I can connect with that need help in reaching their own fitness goals?"

Once they give you a name, make sure to ask how they are connected to the person and the best way to reach them so you can make a smooth connection.

The second way is through a cold referral. A cold referral is when you request referrals from people you have *not* worked with in the past. This may seem a bit more challenging, but below is an easy and disarming approach that you can take with family, friends or coworkers:

"I have a weekly client slot that recently opened up and I'm looking for clients that have concrete fitness goals they would like to achieve. This could be losing a certain amount of weight, or even gaining muscle mass. I've helped many people reach their goals, and I love the challenge. Do you know anyone who has had trouble reaching their goals that would benefit from a *free session* with me?"

Client referrals are among the most powerful tools in growing your personal training business. However, most personal trainers do not receive referrals because they *do not* ask for them. Congratulations on being the exception.

Testimonials and success stories

Testimonials and success stories are quotes and anecdotes specific to your client's health successes. To receive a testimonial or success story, you'll approach clients the same way that you approached them about referrals. When requesting testimonials and success stories, you generally ask clients who you've worked with for at least 1 to 2 months.

For example, you can say, "You've been doing so well with your health. You've lost 20 lbs. in five weeks by consistently exercising and reducing the amount of calories you consume. I respect your commitment and I'd appreciate a quote from you to put on my website."

Remember that your client won't always say yes and provide you with success stories or testimonials. Clients may be taken aback by your request, and you need to be empathetic to their choice. However, if you don't ask for success stories and testimonials, you definitely won't receive them. So find the courage and ask.

Ramping-up your schedule

If you don't have enough clients or are just getting into personal training, there are many activities that can help ramp-up your schedule. I've discussed a few of these ideas in previous sections and I'll expand (below) with additional ideas to help you succeed.

Group Training – An effective activity to increase the amount of money you make in one session, as well as increasing the number of prospective one-on-one clients you work with.

Free Sessions – Providing free sessions are an effective method of filling your schedule, showcasing your skills to prospects and testing your business ideas (strategy). Free sessions are used to give prospects a small amount of value so they are enticed to work with you.

Establish a Community Presence – Your brand will grow in direct proportion to the effort you put into it. If you only personal train in one location, it's difficult for your brand to grow quickly. There are many activities to increase your community presence such as to network with other health professionals, write a blog post for an established health professional, volunteer at fitness events, or create an email subscription list where people can sign up for frequent newsletters on your website and you promote your business by delivering value through health tips and tricks.

You are an Expert – According to the Merriam Webster Dictionary, the definition of "expert" is "having, involving, or displaying special skill or knowledge derived from training or experience." To be an expert, you don't need to know everything in a specific area (i.e. anatomy, program creation, etc.). Even top professionals in any field continue to expand their knowledge base. Your knowledge and experience will already put you in the category of being an expert. The average person will most likely not have the knowledge and skill that you already have from pursuing personal training. You are an expert, so promote yourself as an expert. You can do this with activities such as providing health education at local businesses, creating your own blog, or partnering with professionals offering accompanying services (i.e. a yoga instructor or a nutritionist).

Create a Network – Building a fitness network group is a simple way to build your brand and promote yourself as the expert you are. The network group can be a digital forum where you discuss fitness-related topics online or it can be an in-person meet-up group to get more social interaction.

Social Media Promotion – Every independent personal trainer and gym owner needs to frequently post pictures and videos to social media. Promote. Promote. Promote on social media. More people are spending an increasing amount of their time on social media, so having a social media presence is a must. For all personal trainer employees, most gyms don't allow you to take pictures inside their gyms and post it to your personal social media; however, if you can, do it.

Review Websites – In addition to creating a business website, it's beneficial to establish yourself on review-based websites as they act like referral systems. Some of the best review-based websites to join are LinkedIn, Yelp and TripAdvisor. Ask your clients to review your skills on these websites and share their success stories.

Medical Referral Program – Partner with local doctors, nutritionists, chiropractors and physical therapists. How does this work? Many times health insurance companies will only cover so much of a recovery program (i.e. physical therapy) or a patient is strong enough to leave a physical therapist's care but needs ongoing rehabilitation and support. If you have an established partnership with a physical therapist, you can be the patient's successful transition into a fitness program as a client.

Past Clients – In order to grow, you may need to reach out to past clients. It's beneficial to reach out to all past clients, whether it's just to check in or to ask them to return to training. When you reach out to past clients, they'll have the following thought, "I'm not even this person's client anymore and they're still asking how my health is. They really care about me." Establish strong bonds, increase your value, and increase your success.

Offer an Affiliate Program – Affiliate programs are ways for your brand to get affordable marketing through small partnerships. You allow people to market for you (digital, physical) and if they bring in leads for your business, you pay the affiliate with money or a service discount. Affiliate programs have been highly effective to grow large companies such as Lululemon and Amazon.

Distribute Collateral Material – Collateral material is a fancy term for documentation. Create physical collateral material such as a flyer, pricing handouts, business cards, and direct mailers. Most companies are moving towards digital marketing, so when prospects can hold something physical in their hands it provides an additional connection with the prospect.

More success ideas

There are many ways to make money in the fitness industry. Throughout this book, we've discussed activities that help boost your in-person personal training business. However, there are other ways to make money in the fitness industry.

Options for multiple income streams

So, you're thinking of online personal training? Online training is a good avenue to fill your schedule, especially at time slots that are usually difficult to fill. Online personal training usually puts you in touch with clients all over the world, and you generally work for a reduced price for multiple reasons – people expect cheaper services online and other countries' average personal training prices are lower than in the US.

This can help fill up your schedule (for a time) and can assist you because you can personal train from anywhere. However, it's difficult to assess your client's movement and effectively communicate, which are activities that typically increase your value.

Usually online training happens for two reasons: When a client you already work with in-person is away and you personal train them via a webcam or video call (short time period); or, the more frequent reason is to sign up for an online service who you pay to provide clients and the video conferencing software.

Why would you train online? To fill your schedule, increase your online brand presence, make additional money, and iterate on your brand and services.

An additional method to create multiple income streams, is to expand your fitness product sales with activities such as selling nutritional supplements. Supplement sales can be a lucrative source of income if set up properly.

Moreover, as a fitness professional, you can receive reduced-priced fitness clothes at stores like Lululemon. This doesn't bring in revenue, but it can reduce your business expenditures.

For example, Lululemon has two programs in the United States:

1. Once you prove you're a personal trainer, they provide ~10% discount on clothes;
2. If you have a large enough community presence, you can be a brand ambassador. To become a brand ambassador, Lululemon employees will attend your group fitness class or visit your business to confirm attendance and fitness style. If approved, the company will give you a discount on store purchases and give you free branded clothing

(~$1,000 at Lululemon). This is a great deal for a personal trainer because fitness clothes can be expensive.

BONUS SUCCESS CHECKLISTS

BONUS: Personal Trainer Success Checklist

Astronauts, doctors, teachers, and many other professionals, create checklists to make sure they'll be successful at their jobs. Personal trainers should create checklists so they can also be successful. Over the last ten years, I've created a checklist that will help you increase your success as a personal trainer. Print this list and keep it with you. Soon enough, you'll know the list by heart and will even update it to your individual situation.

I'm giving you my success checklist to eliminate the experience and knowledge gap so that you can be successful immediately. The personal trainer success checklist has the following content:

- Daily checklist – Simple tricks to make you successful every day
- Attire – How to dress for your profession
- Exercise equipment – Suggested equipment used by most trainers, separated into Basic, Intermediate, and Advanced tools
- Non-exercise materials – Suggested material to carry with you as you work, separated into Necessary, Prepared, and Client Compassion items

Personal Trainer Success Checklist Example:

BONUS: Personal Training SUCCESS Checklist

DAILY CHECKLIST

- Confirm appointment with clients prior to first session
- Smile and say hello to everyone
- Business cards
- Business flyers

APPROPRIATE ATTIRE

- ***Branded t-shirt*** - if you work for a gym, they will most likely give you a branded t-shirt or top. If you're an independent Trainer or if you work for a gym and you're exercising, where branded clothing that has your business name, personal name, phone number, email address or website. All of this information is helpful so the prospect can contact you even if they don't meet you in person

- ***Exercise clothing*** – dress the part. Being successful at marketing is creating your individual brand, which begins with how you dress. If you don't look like a Personal Trainer, your prospect pool will diminish

- ***Athletic shoes*** – aim for comfort, because you'll be standing for hours each day

To be a successful personal trainer, you have to work at it. You will not be gifted a successful career, you have to take every opportunity to excel. I've created a Sales Checklist that will help increase the number of sales you make (assessed weekly):

BONUS: Sales Checklist

- Get one referral, testimonial, success story or digital review
- Contact five current clients to help improve their experience

- Contact two prospects who haven't been converted into clients
- Get five new prospects
- Sell two new session bundles

Once you've built a successful foundation, the chapter that will continue to help you, and in which you'll spend the most time reviewing, is this one — Keep Your Momentum. The ideas presented may seem simple, but their implementation and maintenance are complex and crucial.

Measure everything in your business, have flexibility so that you can iterate quickly, make your clients happy and then use their positive stories (testimonials, reviews, success stories) to help increase your business.

Continue your journey and create a successful future...

Chapter Nine

Your Future

*"Combine your natural ability with a mission to help people
and you will have a rich, fulfilling life."*
-Bryan Krahn-

The Vision — The Future

He was on the edge, the cliff dropped away suddenly. Luke started teetering forward, the magnetism of the height drawing him forward — but as he stared down into the depths, a stepping stone appeared... then another and another. Eventually, they joined together to form a bridge and Luke could walk over to the other side. Just before he stepped onto the lush grass, he looked back. There were others behind him, stepping on each stepping stone. They were crossing the bridge. They looked confident... they looked like they knew what they were doing and where they were going. Luke woke up with a start — he knew the way forward.

Over the last couple of years, Ted's mentorship had been a guiding force in Luke's life and saved him years of stress, confusion, and failure. He had given Luke a new appreciation for his career, his services, for himself, and for mentorship.

With Ted's guidance, Luke had built a successful independent personal training business, and he also played an integral role in Ted's gym as one of his top trainers. Luke had added to his certifications, had trained hundreds of clients, had coached trainers at big box gyms across the country and given talks at universities and fitness conventions. He had branched out into the corporate world and worked with companies to improve their staff health and wellness. The value that he brought to his clients' lives and to others had brought value to his bank account. Luke was successful, but he wanted to push forward in his growth, not only as a personal trainer and coach — but in business and in his character. He called Ted.

"Hi Luke, how's it going?" Ted answered his phone.

"I've been thinking, Ted. You know your system that you used to coach me in business and personal training? The steps that we took to build my business?" Luke sounded excited, "Well, what about if we use your process to develop an online educational platform that integrates personal training, life values, life coaching and business skills?"

"That's brilliant, Luke! I think that's a great idea. We can make a difference in so many people's lives through reaching them online. I'm very interested. We have our gym staff meeting this afternoon, bring your ideas and we can work on them. That sounds awesome!"

When Luke put the phone down, he smiled. He had that sense of excitement brewing — it was time for the next adventure.

***

> "The most dangerous poison is the feeling of achievement. The antidote is to every evening think, what can be done better tomorrow."
> -Ingvar Kamprad-

You've made it so far. Whether you're a prospective or experienced personal trainer, you've just boosted your knowledge by years. You've identified your values, needs, and goals. You've explored your fears, which led to understanding the areas of improvement. You've identified and outlined the missing pieces in your business, such as creating a better brand, creating more value through sales and marketing, or updating your assessment questions.

You were given tools to use in business, sales, marketing, and health programs, and then you expanded on these tools by integrating them into your daily life. Together we discussed setting up your business, kicking off sales and marketing, how to get more clients, how to walk through a session, success tips for a training session, and how to make more money.

The common questions that plague personal trainers such as, "How do I get my first client(s)?", "How do I sell?", and "How do I create value for my clients?" were answered. You were also provided with ideas for increasing your prices, getting passive income, receiving testimonials, asking for referrals, and making more money in general. Additionally, you learned the iteration life cycle and full-service personal training basics along the way. As you have applied yourself throughout this book, your business has gained so much value. You have also come to understand that the role of the personal trainer is an honorable and central place to be. That's why so much emphasis was placed on the personal connection and relationship-building aspect of personal training. You're not just providing workout programs for clients. You care for your clients; you integrate health into their lives and facilitate lifestyle changes; you coach, you counsel, you cheer and you motivate. You are bringing value and you enable your clients to achieve what they can't do on their own. You are a life-changer.

Your future

How can you continue to be successful? It's beneficial to go through the book's activities every six months as your goals and needs change. Growth is a continuous endeavor and a surefire way to increase your value.

The goal is to stay humble, understanding that there's always something to work on; focus on how you can better serve your clients; continue learning about your business, your clients, and yourself; and most importantly keep a positive attitude.

You have learned a lot throughout this book and it is your goal to succeed. Why will you succeed? You will succeed as a personal trainer because you'll continue to build value in your business every day, in each interaction, through every activity.

Congratulations on undertaking this journey towards success and I am thankful to have been a part of it. However, your journey does not end here — this is just the beginning.

In order to achieve something you've never done before, you must be willing to become somebody you've never been before. Keep growing and moving forward towards your success.

If you would like more information, materials, tools and additional services. You can find it at my website - www.MakeMoneyPersonalTraining.com

Appendix: Exercise & Activities Checklists

Chapter Three - Facing Your Fears

EXERCISE	DATE COMPLETED
Follow the 7 steps outlined in the Fear Setting exercise.	

Chapter Four - Laying Your Foundation

EXERCISE	DATE COMPLETED
Follow the 4 steps outlined in the Partial Success exercise.	
Follow the 5 steps outlined in the Cost of Inaction exercise.	
Follow the 7 steps outlined in the S.M.A.R.T. Goals exercise.	
Follow the 4 steps outlined in the Vision Board exercise.	

Chapter Six — Set Up Your Success

ACTIVITY	DATE COMPLETED
Choose a certification to acquire.	
Select where you want to work.	
Create a 6-month calendar for all the provided exercise templates and any additional exercise templates you created yourself.	
Select your niche.	
Select your preferred trainer type.	
Select your business location.	
Select your pricing model.	
Create your business plan.	
List the type of funding you will prioritize.	
Complete each task in the successful business operations section and develop all branded tools from the previous section.	
Write rules for yourself and your clients.	

Set up your digital marketing, reach out for referrals, and develop all tools from the previous section.	
Write your own daily brand checklist.	

Chapter Seven - Building Your Business Success

ACTIVITY	DATE COMPLETED
Write two conversations, directing a chatty and quiet client on the importance of regular communication.	
Record activities that will turn you into a full-service personal trainer.	
Make a list of at least three marketing ideas to help acquire your first clients.	
With respect to your niche and target client, write a pitch outline.	
Using the list of objections, select one and write out a complete transcript example where you answer their objections using the success path (steps 1 – 6). Bonus points for writing a transcript for all the aforementioned objections and for practicing objection conversations with a friend or coworker.	

If you're an experienced personal trainer, review your lost opportunities from the past 1, 3, 6, or 12 months. If possible, identify negative patterns and plan how you will change that habit in the future using the outlined pitch and objection handling techniques.	

Recommended Reading

Personal Training Books:

- Boyle, Michael. *Advances in Functional Training: Training Techniques for Coaches, Personal Trainers and Athletes.* BookBaby, 2012.
- *Essentials of Strength Training and Conditioning* (NSCA book)
- Chek, Paul. *How to Eat, Move and Be Healthy: Your Personalized 4-Step Guide to Looking and Feeling from inside Out.* C.H.E.K Institute, 2004.
- Cook, Gray. *Movement: Functional Movement Systems: Screening, Assessment, Corrective Strategies.* BookBaby, 2010.
- Cook, Gray. *Athletic Body in Balance.* 2003.
- Perry, Jacquelin, et al. *Gait Analysis: Normal and Pathological Function.* Slack, 2010.
- Williams, Roger J. *Biochemical Individuality: the Basis for the Genetotrophic Concept:* Keats Publishing, 1998.

Business Books:

- Collins, James C. *Good to Great: Why Some Companies Make the Leap ... and Others Don't.* HarperBusiness, 2001.
- Duhigg, Charles. *The Power of Habit: Why We Do What We Do and How to Change.* Random House, 2013.
- Ries, Eric. *The Lean Startup.* Summaries.com, 2013.
- Tzu, Sun. *Sun Tzu: the Art of War.* Everyman's Library, 2018.

Sales and Marketing Books:

- Baer, Jay. *Hug Your Haters: How to Embrace Complaints and Keep Your Customers.* Portfolio/PENGUIN, 2016.
- Baer, Jay. *Youtility: Why Smart Marketing Is about Help Not Hype.* Portfolio, 2014.
- Berger, Jonah. *Contagious: Why Things Catch On.* Simon & Schuster, 2013.
- Carnegie, Dale. *How to Win Friends and Influence People: a Condensation from the Book.* Snowball Pub., 2010.
- Klaff, Oren. *Pitch Anything: an Innovative Method for Presenting, Persuading and Winning the Deal.* McGraw-Hill, 2011.
- Levinson, Jay Conrad. *Guerilla Marketing*: Computer Press, 2009.
- Pink, Daniel H. *To Sell is Human: the Surprising Truth about Persuading, Convincing, and Influencing Others.* Canongate Books Ltd, 2018.
- Schaefer, Mark W. *The Content Code: Six Essential Strategies for Igniting Your Content, Your Marketing, and Your Business.* Schaefer Marketing Solutions, 2015.
- Sheridan, Marcus. *They Ask You Answer: a Revolutionary Approach to Inbound Sales, Content Marketing, and Today's Digital Consumer.* Wiley, 2017.

Resources and References

http://www.exrx.net/ - comprehensive exercise prescription

Chapter One

- "Claus Moser, Baron Moser." *Wikiquote.* en.wikiquote.org/wiki/Claus_Moser,_Baron_Moser.
- "Personal Trainer Salary | How Much Do Trainers Make?" *National Federation of Professional Trainers.* www.nfpt.com/personal-trainer-salary.
- "Personal Trainer." *Wikipedia.* en.wikipedia.org/wiki/Personal_trainer.
- "Personal Trainer Salaries." *Personal Trainer Salaries by Education, Experience, Location and More - Salary.com.* www1.salary.com/Personal-Trainer-Salary.html.

Chapter Two

- "If Your WHY Is Strong Enough You Will Figure out the HOW!" *Bill Walsh® - America's Business Expert.* billwalshblog.com/if-your-why-is-strong-enough-you-will-figure-out-the-how/.
- Jakes, TD. "17 Quotes That Will Help You Discover Your Life's Purpose."*Oprah.com.* www.oprah.com/spirit/quotes-to-help-you-find-your-lifes-purpose--inspirational-quotes/
- **Chapter Three**
- "Mandela, Nelson."*BrainyQuote.* https://www.brainyquote.com/authors/nelson_mandela
- H.P. Lovecraft. *BrainyQuote.* https://www.brainyquote.com/quotes/h_p_lovecraft_676245

Chapter Four

- "Carol Burnett Quotes." *BrainyQuote.* www.brainyquote.com/authors/carol_burnett.
- "Top 10Earl NightingaleQuotes." *BrainyQuote.* www.brainyquote.com/lists/authors/top_10_earl_nighti ngale_quotes.

Chapter Five

- Maraboli, Steve. "Quotes About Tools (68 Quotes)." *(68 Quotes).* www.goodreads.com/quotes/tag/tools.
- "Chawla, Kalpana." *BrainyQuote.* www.brainyquote.com/search_results?q=Kalpana.
- Peters, Tom. "50 Amazing Personal Branding Quotes You Need to Know." *navid moazzez.* https://navidmoazzez.com/best-personal-branding-quotes/

Chapter Six

- USA stats. "Obesity and Overweight."*Centers for Disease Control and Prevention.* https://www.cdc.gov/nchs/fastats/obesity-overweight.htm
- Soroush, Abdolkarim. *BrainyQuote.* www.brainyquote.com/search_results?q=++Abdolkarim +Soroush.
- Carmack, John. *BrainyQuote.* www.brainyquote.com/search_results?q=+John+Carma ck.

Chapter Seven

- Freitas, Ryan. Warren, Renée. "101 Best Inspirational Quotes For Entrepreneurs." *Business Insider,* Business

Insider, 7 Sept. 2013, www.businessinsider.com/101-best-inspirational-quotes-for-entrepreneurs-2013-9.

- Blakely,Sara. Warren, Renée. "101 Best Inspirational Quotes For Entrepreneurs." *Business Insider*, Business Insider, 7 Sept. 2013, www.businessinsider.com/101-best-inspirational-quotes-for-entrepreneurs-2013-9.

Chapter Eight

- Powell, Colin. *BrainyQuote*, www.brainyquote.com/search_results?q=colin+Powel.
- Johnny Cash. Walter, Ekaterina. "30 Powerful Quotes on Failure." *Forbes*, Forbes Magazine, 20 Sept. 2015, www.forbes.com/sites/ekaterinawalter/2013/12/30/30-powerful-quotes-on-failure/#120b7b4b24bd.
- **Chapter Nine**
- Krahn,Bryan. "15 Best Motivational Quotes for Fitness Professionals." *AFPA fitness*. https://www.afpafitness.com/blog/15-best-motivational-quotes-for-fitness-professionals
- Kampar, Ingvar. *Startupquote*. http://startupquote.com/post/12661360913

About the Author

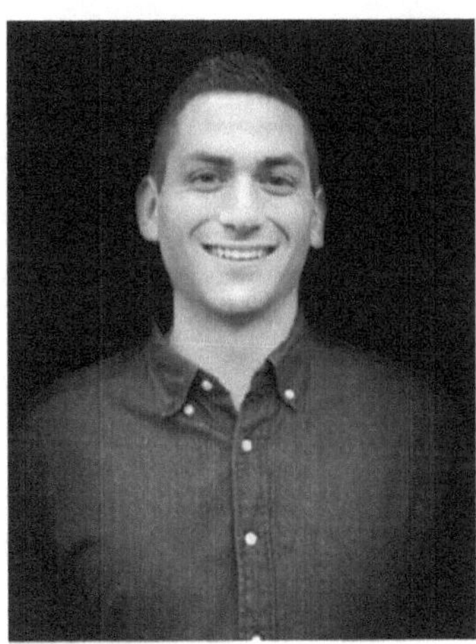

Jared Garcia has a degree in Exercise Biology from the University of California, Davis, and has been certified as a personal trainer with NSCA-CSCS, TRX, Z-Health, CHEK Holistic Lifestyle Coach, FMS, USA Weightlifting, and ACE.

Throughout his personal training career, he's worked in big box gyms, small private gyms, universities, physical therapy clinics, with sports teams, and he's opened his own independent training business. He's taught large and small group training, one-on-one personal training, personal training program creation classes, personal training exercise selection and equipment selection classes, helped launch new group training programs and has consulted on health-related software apps.

Additionally, he's designed, prototyped and built fitness products; as well as created a health blog focused on exercise and nutrition. Jared is the CEO of MMPT (Make Money Personal Training), an online education platform designed to help personal trainers of all experience levels find success ... and earn more money.

Contact the Author

Throughout my personal training career, I've assisted many personal trainers to achieve their goals in the various areas of their professional and personal training businesses. I enjoy helping personal trainers of any experience level discover the value that they can bring, resulting in them achieving greater levels of success. As such, if you have questions or feedback please reach out to me using the following email address:

Jared@MMPT.co

Additionally, find more information for a personal training success course using the following website:

MakeMoneyPersonalTraining.com

I look forward to chatting with you soon,

Jared Garcia